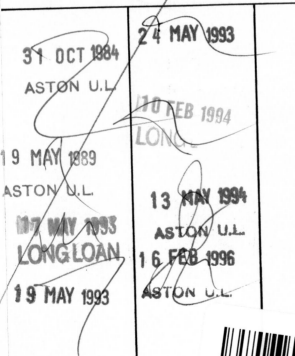

This book is due for return not later than the last date
stamped below, unless recalled sooner.

Prevention of Spina Bifida and Other Neural Tube Defects

Based on a Workshop sponsored by Rybar Laboratories Ltd. and held at The Lygon Arms, Broadway, Worcestershire, England, 3–6 October, 1982

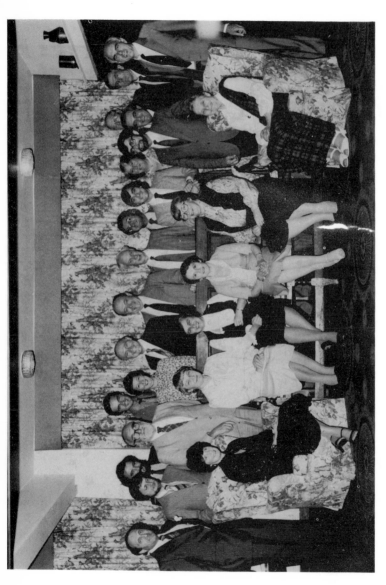

Members of the Workshop, Observers, and their Wives. Back row (left to right): K. Michael Laurence, Chris J. Schorer, Colin Tudge, Hubert Campbell, Paedar Kirke, Mary J. Seller, Norman C. Nevin, John Dobbing, Richard W. Smithells, Andrew Tisman, Ron Akehurst, Jean Sands, Nicholas Wald, Donald J. Naismith, Felix Beck, John H. Edwards, Ian Leck. Front Row: Mrs Schorer, Mrs Smithells, Mrs Beck, Mrs Nevin, Mrs Laurence, Mrs Campbell.

Prevention of Spina Bifida and Other Neural Tube Defects

Edited by

John Dobbing
Department of Child Health,
The Medical School
University of Manchester,
England

1983

Academic Press
A Subsidiary of Harcourt Brace Jovanovich, Publishers
London   New York
Paris   San Diego   San Francisco   São Paulo
Sydney   Tokyo   Toronto

ACADEMIC PRESS INC. (LONDON) LTD.
24/28 Oval Road
London NW1

United States Edition published by
ACADEMIC PRESS INC.
111 Fifth Avenue
New York, New York 10003

British Library Cataloguing in Publication Data

Prevention of spina bifida and other neural tube defects.
1. Spina bifida – Congresses
I. Dobbing, J.
618.9′27′3043   RJ496.574

ISBN 0-12-218860-8
LCCCN 83-070170

Typeset by Oxford Verbatim Limited
Printed and bound in Great Britain by
T. J. Press (Padstow) Ltd., Cornwall

Contributors

R. L. Akehurst, *Economic Aspects of Clinical Practice, Institute of Social and Economic Research, University of York, Heslington, York YO1 5DD.*

Felix Beck, *Department of Anatomy, The Medical School, University of Leicester, University Road, Leicester LE1 7RH.*

Hubert Campbell, *Department of Medical Statistics, Welsh National School of Medicine, Heath Park, Cardiff CF4 4XN.*

J. A. Davis,* *Department of Paediatrics, Level 8, Addenbrooke's Hospital, Hills Rd., Cambridge CB2 2QQ.*

John Dobbing, *Department of Child Health, University of Manchester, The Medical School, Oxford Road, Manchester M13 9PT.*

J. H. Edwards, *Department of Medical Genetics, Oxfordshire A.H.A. (Teaching), Old Road, Headington, Oxford OX3 7LE.*

Cynthia A. Iles,* *Community Medicine Section, Medical Unit, University College Hospital Medical School, London.*

Nansi E. James,* *Department of Child Health, Welsh National School of Medicine, Heath Park, Cardiff CF4 4XN.*

Peadar N. Kirke, *The Medico-Social Research Board, 73 Lower Baggot Street, Dublin 2, Eire.*

K. M. Laurence, *Department of Paediatric Research, Welsh National School of Medicine, Heath Park, Cardiff CF4 4XN.*

Ian Leck, *Department of Community Medicine, University of Manchester, The Medical School, Oxford Road, Manchester M13 9PT.*

D. J. Naismith, *Department of Food Science and Nutrition, Queen Elizabeth College, University of London, Atkin Building, Campden Hill, London W8 7AH.*

Norman C. Nevin, *Department of Medical Genetics, The Queen's University of Belfast, Institute of Clinical Science, Grosvenor Road, Belfast BT12 6BJ, Northern Ireland.*

C. J. Schorah, *Department of Chemical Pathology, The Old Medical School, Thoresby Place, Leeds LS2 9NL.*

Mary J. Seller, *Paediatric Research Unit, 7th Floor, Guy's Tower, Guy's Hospital, London SE1 9RT.*

I. M. Sharman,* *Dunn Nutritional Laboratory, University of Cambridge, Milton Road, Cambridge CB4 1XJ.*

R. W. Smithells, *University of Leeds, Department of Paediatrics, 27 Blundell St., Leeds LS1 3ET.*

Thane Toe,* *Department of Human Nutrition, London School of Hygiene and Tropical Medicine, Keppel St., London WC1E 7HT.*

G. R. Wadsworth,* *Department of Human Nutrition, London School of Hygiene and Tropical Medicine, Keppel St., London WC1E 7HT.*

Nicholas Wald, *I.C.R.F. Cancer Epidemiology and Clinical Trials Unit, Gibson Laboratories, The Radcliffe Infirmary, Oxford OX2 6HE.*

* Did not attend the Workshop.

Preface

There are some medical conditions which are so disastrous for the individual and his family as well as for society, not to mention for the attendant doctor, that almost any hint of a solution is eagerly grasped, sometimes long before it emerges from the status of a suggestion into one supported by evidence and proper trial. In these cases everyone involved, including the doctor, is quite reasonably tempted to lower the standard of proof which is normally required before a discovery can be accepted and incorporated into normal practice. Such a condition is spina bifida, and its other related neural tube defects; and such a proposed solution is a preventive one, the credentials of which this book strives to examine.

Lay people, including non-medical scientists, do not always appreciate the extent to which practising doctors find it necessary to act with decision in particular cases, long before proof is available which would be acceptable to other scientific disciplines. Whether the latter like it or not, a doctor's management of his patient can never be restricted by the proper constraints of pure science, except in the sense that real science, taking into account all aspects of a problem as it must, might not always impose such constraints. The obstacles to unimpeachable proof in matters such as these are many, but they do not acquit the doctor of the duty to strive to overcome them, even when he knows that proof can never be completely attained. At the very least he should be fully conscious of the extent to which the knowledge on which his inevitable current judgements are founded falls short of the ideal. Anything less would not be honest.

It was in this spirit that a Workshop was organized which provided the material for this book. The central question, arising from a series of preliminary findings in several centres in the British Isles, was whether periconceptional supplementation of the maternal diet with certain vitamins could prevent neural tube defects in the offspring. The witnesses assembled to testify were representative of all those who, at that point in time (October

1982), had produced evidence. Those of their colleagues and co-workers who did not take part are all acknowledged, either formally by co-authorship, or by implication in the bibliography.

In order to appreciate the novel way in which the knowledge, findings and opinions recorded here were distilled, it will be helpful to understand something of the organization of the Workshop. This was the second occasion of its type, and was organized in an identical manner to the first, which was described in the first monograph (1) as follows:

Six authors were chosen several months before the meeting, each being asked to write papers setting out their own attitudes to the question. Authors were chosen for their authority and because of their own major participation in the findings so far. Each paper was then precirculated to each of the other five, as well as to six other people who had contributed just as substantially to the subject, or who possessed key expertise in related disciplines. All twelve people were asked to write a critique of all the papers, and these too were then circulated to all the participants, several weeks before the Workshop was held. By the time we gathered together for the Workshop, therefore, all the papers had already been assimilated and so had all the immediate reactions to them. Furthermore several of the original papers had undergone further modification in the light of the comments received, bearing in mind that those comments had been written out, in a considered manner, with references where appropriate.

The Workshop itself consisted exclusively of discussion. The conventional format, in which speakers often use most of the available time giving their talks, followed by a few barely considered questions masquerading as a discussion, any meaningful debate being largely confined to the corridors outside or the coffee room, was avoided.

The discussion was not recorded. No one was inhibited by microphones or the turning of reels of tape, and it has, therefore, not been necessary to transcribe the endless, tedious colloquialisms which occasionally mar reports of this kind.

More importantly there was deliberately no attempt to arrive at a consensus. Striving for agreement almost always leads to a lowest common denominator in which there can be no proper exposure of important areas of difference which exist very productively amongst the students of most important research topics.

It can be said at once that the main design itself was enormously successful, particularly from the point of view of the participants. It is probably true to say that no one came through the experience without undergoing some fairly substantial change. In this sense the interests of our subject have been well served and we have ourselves been educated.

Compiling a publication so that you, the reader, may participate in our pleasure and purification has been a much harder task.

First, most of the original papers have been substantially modified without your having been able to participate in the refining process which brought this about, an experience which was of such benefit to those of us who were there. It may be some compensation that the final versions reproduced here have all passed through a sort of peer-review system unlike most others. They represent their authors' very considered views in the face of criticism by representatives of most contrary opinion.

Secondly, time was made available for the original commentaries to be modified where necessary after the discussions, and a selection of these is presented rather in the form of a children's scrapbook at the end of each paper and at the end of the book. By definition this makes for a "scrappy" presentation but we could think of no alternative. No editor could have done justice to a summary of everyone's attitudes, and even an edited transcription of the verbal discussion would have risked, as does sometimes happen, the conversion of serious endeavour into farce.

You, the reader, are now left to find your own way through the argument just as we, the participants, had to do at Broadway.

The present Workshop was an exact copy of the first. As before, and as was expected, this resulting monograph does not contain any consensus statement of the present view. None such exists. The reader is, as previously, quite properly put to the inconvenience of drawing his own conclusions.

The first two chapters are concerned with the contribution of experimental, laboratory research to the immediate question. Mary Seller writes about whole animal experiments and how these may illuminate our subject. Felix Beck introduces the ways in which whole embryo culture may provide a short cut to solving some of the remaining problems. As Chairman and Editor, I found both these propositions most convincing, a view which was only partly shared by some. It has always seemed to me that clinicians (though not necessarily those represented here) are often far from consistent in their attitudes to animal experiments in medical research. They sometimes decry the usefulness of animal experiments to human medical practice, while at the same time embracing those same animals when it comes to supporting their own emotionally held convictions, even though these latter may be so self-evident that they scarcely need support anyway! (Examples in paediatrics are the superiority of breast-feeding, and the boundless benefits of mother–infant bonding in the first minutes after birth.) I think my colleagues' frequent mistrust of animal experiments stems from the deficiencies of their (and my) medical scientific education. We are taught about only one species, as if it were unique. We also too readily see it as our target to find animal "models" which mimic human disease in all respects, even though human diseases are rarely so stereotyped and such models scarcely exist. Of course if such a model can be devised it can be useful, but the main rôle of animal work is to be able ethically and experimentally to examine key links in an aetiological chain, and to do so in a very much shorter time than could ever be done in our own, slowly growing species. Total matching to a human disease is not required for expressing, for example, the general mix of genetic and environmental influences on an outcome; or to disentangle whether one vitamin out of a mixture is active, either alone or by interaction with the others, in preventing a biological catastrophe. In short, we doctors do not easily acknowledge how much of our current clinical practice owes to painstaking work with experimental animals. The fact that much research in *developing* animals is badly extrapolated to man because it ignores the different rates of growth and development and the different stages of maturity at birth between species; or sometimes uses quite unrealistic doses of assayed substances compared with those obtaining in humans; or forgets to define the known absolute differences which exist between species (differences which diminish the further back one goes into the embryological stages of recapitulation); all these deficiencies tell us more about the experimenter or of some of his clinician-judges than about their intrinsic usefulness. Thus Felix Beck has cogently argued the great *advantage* of embryo culture in separating the mother from the embryo, a separation which others were tempted to deem a *disadvantage*.

After the first two chapters on experiments in laboratory animals come three on the experiments in humans which have so far been performed on sizeable populations. Dick Smithells very lucidly summarizes the multicentre study in which he and many of his colleagues looked at the efficacy of a proprietary multivitamin cocktail, administered before conception and for the first weeks of pregnancy, in avoiding the expected number of neural tube defects in a population of mothers at high risk. He acknowledges the deficiencies of his experimental design, to the satisfaction of the great majority of the participants, and comes to the practical conclusion that little further effort need be devoted to substantiating the result. There was some dissent from this latter view, notably but not exclusively from Nick Wald, and the argument is set out in the pages that follow.

Concurrently with the above study, Michael Laurence and his colleagues were examining the possible prophylactic effects of general dietary advice and, more specifically, of a fairly large supplement of folic acid to high risk mothers. Their conclusions, at their simplest, lean towards the view that folic acid is likely to be the key active constituent in the diet, or in Smithells' cocktail. There was a large number of criticisms of Laurence's experimental design, which was defended on two main grounds: that a massive study in a large human population is extremely difficult to do tidily; and that if their findings are positive and striking, in spite of an untidy performance, they are likely to have even more meaning. The argument revealed in the pages that follow is, like that for other chapters, only the tip of an iceberg, its main sub-marine bulk being submerged beneath the threshold of visibility in the many amendments made to the chapter as the result of Workshop discussion, both precirculated and verbal, before it reached its final form.

Northern Ireland is one of the areas of Great Britain where the number of cases of neural tube defects is particularly high. Norman Nevin contributes a chapter which puts the particular problems of his own area and his own success in dealing with them in the context of the general question.

In the last chapter Ian Leck presents a most comprehensive review of the ways in which his own discipline of epidemiology can, in his view, provide clues to the causation of neural tube defects. He concludes that besides high risks in, for example, the offspring of diabetics, the risks are probably increased by folate deficiency and possibly by zinc deficiency. Even though constitutional factors also exert their influence, that of the diet and other variables in the environment allows the hope that we may have the capacity to intervene. In an Appendix, Leck and his colleagues describe a study of patients in a London obstetric clinic in which it was found that blood folate tended to be relatively low in mothers of malformed children, and also in the social classes and months in which the risks of developing neural tube defects seem to be especially high.

Finally there are two short Appendixes contributed by two of the "discussants". Ron Akehurst is a health economist who was invited because we wished to have some idea of the economic implications of our subject. If we did not get everything we asked of him it may have been partly because we were less aware than we should have been that his subject is at least as complex as our own, and with an even more bewildering set of unmeasured, or even unmeasurable variables. Nick Wald was a very valued participant in the discussion, partly because of his membership of a team appointed by the Medical Research Council to consider the usefulness of a further extensive trial, but mainly because of his much greater, and very considered reservations in interpreting the results to date. His views gave rise to a longer discussion than is evident from the material published here, since attempts by everyone to shift each other's opinions were strenuous. For my own part I was left with a rather platitudinous quotation from my Preface to the previous monograph (1): "There is absolutely no substitute for striving endlessly for scientific purity; but it is anti-scientific not to recognize the artistry involved in visualising an entire painting from only a tiny fragment of the canvas."

I wish to express my enormous gratitude to all who took part in the Workshop. The amount of hard work in the months leading up to it, and the eventual intense and lengthy sessions demanded a great deal more from the participants than does the usual form of medical scientific meeting. They found some reward in their quite evident enjoyment of the occasion, and I hope they will find still more in this memorial to their efforts. The Workshop design is still an experiment of my own in which they very generously took part. We met in great cultural and material comfort in the centuries-old Lygon Arms in Broadway, Worcestershire, in countryside amongst the finest and most historic our nation has to offer. My secretary, Mrs Irene Warrington, worked tirelessly at the immense task of producing and circulating almost seven thousand copies of typewritten sheets; and my wife, Dr Jean Sands, was an invaluable help in managing the day-to-day affairs of the actual meeting.

I would also like to place on record my appreciation of the continuing help of Action Research for the Crippled Child (The National Fund for Research into Crippling Diseases). They were not asked to contribute towards the costs of the Workshop, but their generous and continuing support of much of the research reported here, and also of my own position, has played a key rôle in making it possible. We can only hope that their enormous investment in the prevention of handicap will be successful in this area as in others, and that they in their turn will continue to be supported around the country by ordinary people who, after all, have considerable faith in us.

The entire cost of the meeting was borne by Rybar Laboratories Ltd. Their Managing Director, Ronald Levin, F.P.S., responded unhesitatingly at the outset to my importunate request. He read all the precirculated documents personally, and made several significant comments during the run-up period. He explained to us at the last session that his motivation in supporting us was threefold: as a man with some acquaintance of child handicap and the resulting tragedy amongst his close friends, and a consequent desire to help find solutions; as a scientist; and as Managing Director of his company. On behalf of us all I thank him most warmly, and wish him every success in all three capacities.

January 1983

John Dobbing
Hayfield.

1. Dobbing, J., Ed. (1981). "Maternal Nutrition in Pregnancy: Eating for Two?" Academic Press, London.

Contents

Contents

To The National Fund for Research into Crippling Diseases (Action Research for the Crippled Child) to whom the Editor owes much for their continuing help, and who supported a great deal of the research described and discussed here.

Maternal Nutritional Factors and
Neural Tube Defects in Experimental Animals

MARY J. SELLER

Paediatric Research Unit,
Guy's Hospital Medical School,
London

A significant advance in the primary prevention of neural tube defects (NTD) may well be the finding that periconceptional supplementation with physiological doses of multivitamins is associated with a markedly reduced recurrence of NTD in "at risk" women (40, 41, 42). The implication of this work is that a deficiency of one or more of a number of vitamins mediated through the mother somehow contributes to the cause of NTD in the fetus.

It had long been thought, using evidence from epidemiological and family studies, that the cause of NTD was multifactorial with two components interacting – a genetic predisposition triggered by an environmental factor or factors (4). How many genes are involved and what traits they influence have never been determined, but there have been numerous suggestions as to the precipitating environmental agent; however, none has withstood the test of time and close scrutiny. The suggestion that maternal vitamin deficiency may be implicated (39), followed-up by the clinical trial in humans designed to remedy that deficiency, which has apparently been successful in reducing the number of NTD, means that the identification of the environmental component could now be close at hand.

Notwithstanding, much remains to be determined. The tablet which was administered to the women in the intervention study, Pregnavite forte F® (Bencard), is a compound containing 10 vitamins or co-factors (Table 1).

Mary J. Seller

Table 1. Composition of daily dose of Pregnavite forte
F (Bencard) in 3 tablets compared with United States
Recommended Daily Allowances.

	Pregnavite forte F	US RDA
Vitamin A (IU)	4000	5000
Vitamin D (IU)	400	400
Thiamine (mg)	1·5	1·4
Riboflavin (mg)	1·5	1·5
Pyridoxine (mg)	1	2·6
Nicotinamide (mg)	15	15
Ascorbic acid (mg)	40	80
Folic acid (mg)	0·36	0·80
Iron (mg)	75·6	60
Calcium (mg)	141	1200
Phosphorus (mg)	109	1200

Any one of these, or any combination of more than one, may have been the effective agent. Further, simply to identify a preventive agent, satisfactory though it may be clinically, is insufficient scientifically. It is important that the mechanism by which it acts, and how it interacts with the genetic component are determined, so that the underlying pathogenic process in the production of the lesion may be understood. Animal models of human congenital abnormalities suggest that this is likely to be a very complex matter. For example, the gene–environment interaction in the cause of cleft palate in the mouse has been shown to be extremely intricate (13). While the disadvantage of animal models is that findings in them are not necessarily the same as in man (for example, thalidomide has little effect on mice and rats but is severely teratogenic in man) the great advantage of animals is that they may be manipulated and analysed in ways which humans cannot. In so doing they can reveal information and general principles which may well be applicable to man.

This paper describes what can be learnt from studies in animals which may shed light on any influence that maternal nutritional factors may have in the cause and prevention of NTD.

Firstly, is there any evidence that in animals, deficiency of any of the components of Pregnavite forte F, or any other vitamin, does actually cause NTD?

Deficiencies of many individual vitamins during pregnancy in animals have been shown to have devastating effects on the embryo, and to result in growth retardation, intrauterine death and major congenital abnormalities. All organ systems may be affected, but not necessarily all at one time, and the central nervous system (CNS) may or may not be involved. It was, in fact, the observation that a maternal deficiency of vitamin A was associated with abnormal offspring that founded modern teratology. In 1933, Hale (18) noted that a vitamin A deficient sow produced piglets "without eyeballs", and he subsequently showed that this deficiency could also result in cleft lip, accessory ears, subcutaneous cysts and misplaced kidneys (19, 20). However, vitamin A deficiency has never been observed to cause NTD. Comprehensive studies in vitamin A deficient rats found ocular and urogenital defects (47, 48) and cardiac anomalies (49). Hydrocephalus was observed in neonatal rabbits when the vitamin A deficiency occurred late in gestation (27).

Folic acid deficiency, on the other hand, is a well-known cause of CNS defects as well as other abnormalities. A folic acid deficient diet, together with added 1% succinyl sulphathiazole to inhibit intestinal folic acid synthesis, and $0·5\%$ α methyl pteroyl-glutamic acid (PGA) an antagonist, fed to the pregnant rat, resulted in exencephaly and abnormalities in several other systems (29). The administration of certain folic acid antagonists alone is also effective. Twenty and 50 mg/kg of methotrexate, but not 10 mg/kg, given to the mouse resulted in exencephaly, omphalocoele, ectrodactly and cleft palate (38). Tuchmann-Duplessis *et al.* (43) found that this agent produced CNS abnormalities in rats and cats as well as mice. Another folic acid antagonist, aminopterin, caused CNS defects and eye, tail, extremity and abdominal wall abnormalities in the rat (2).

Of the other vitamins, pyridoxine (B_6) deficiency in rats caused exencephaly, cleft palate, omphalocoele and ectrodactyly (9); vitamin E deficiency produced exencephaly or hydrocephaly in rats (5) but not mice (21); pantothenic acid deficiency caused exencephaly in rats (25); and vitamin B_{12} deficiency in rats resulted in NTD and hydronephrosis (50). But lack of either riboflavin or vitamin D, although causing other abnormalities, did not produce NTD (44, 45). Little is known about the effects of vitamin C deficiency, because most animals synthesize their own. Only man and other primates and the guinea pig require dietary ascorbic acid.

Thus there is definite evidence for deficiencies of maternal nutritional factors causing NTD in animals. Further, in some cases deficiencies of certain vitamins may interact with deficiencies of other substances, for example the simultaneous depletion of both vitamin A and zinc leads to more severe abnormalities in the rat than the lack of either alone (11). Conversely, by the way, the presence of riboflavin will decrease the teratogenic effects of a phenothiazine derivative (22).

Zinc deficiency alone has been suggested as a cause of NTD in man (see Chapters by Nevin and Leck). However, in animals, a lack of zinc is more commonly associated with hydrocephaly. Hurley and Swenerton (24) found no NTD amongst the congenital abnormalities produced by maternal zinc depletion in rats, neither did Dreosti *et al*. (10). Warkany and Petering (46) found only 2% of offspring from zinc depleted mothers with exencephaly, but 20% with hydrocephaly. If the zinc depletion was made to extend for the duration of pregnancy, more offspring had NTD, 11% with exencephaly and 3% with spina bifida. However, hydrocephalus then occurred in 47% of offspring (23). Accompanying anatomical and histological studies led Hurley and Schrader (23) to conclude that the developmental defects of the brain in zinc deficient rats involves primary closure of the aqueduct. Thus the evidence in animals for true NTD being caused by zinc deficiency is suggestive, but other abnormalities of the central nervous system are caused more commonly.

The effects of vitamin excess, too, have been examined in animals. Certain malformations are associated with excess vitamin D (13), vitamin E (28), 6-amino-nicotinamide (8) and vitamin A, but it is only with hypervitaminosis A that NTDs occur. This is of crucial importance in the present context, because it is a potent teratogen of the rodent CNS, and vitamin A is present in Pregnavite forte F. The effect was initially discovered in rats when 35 000 IU given daily from the second to the 16th day of gestation produced exencephaly in 54% of the offspring (6). Subsequently it has been found that both exencephaly and spina bifida, as well as other abnormalities, can be produced consistently by similar doses in the mouse, guinea pig and rabbit (16), hamster (26) and the pig (30). In humans, there is a single report of a woman who took 25 000 IU vitamin A each day for the first 3 months of pregnancy, and double that dose daily thereafter, whose child had urogenital abnormalities (3). The daily dose of vitamin A in Pregnavite forte F is 4000 IU, which is substantially lower than both the teratogenic doses in animals, especially when considered on a dose per body weight basis, and the dose which produced relatively minor defects in man. It is, in fact, similar to the recommended daily intake for women in pregnancy.

The science of teratology flourished in the wake of the tragic consequences of the use of thalidomide. An enormous number of experiments have been performed on the effects of drugs on the developing conceptus. From these studies have emerged some general principles regarding the production of major developmental abnormalities which have implications when considering how maternal nutritional factors may influence NTD in man.

The embryo is only vulnerable to environmental assault for a relatively short time in its prenatal life. Generally, although there are exceptions, no major abnormalities arise if exposure to environmental agents comes before the time of implantation or after the main morphogenetic processes have been completed. The sensitive time is the period of organogenesis. Within that period, the types of abnormalities and the particular organ systems affected differ according to the stage of pregnancy reached when the environmental factors are operative. Each structure has its own critical time of sensitivity, which is usually immediately before, and during, its formation. Thus, hypervitaminosis A affects the rodent CNS around days 7 and 8 of pregnancy, but has no effect on the palate at this time, the critical period for the palate occurs later, at which time the CNS is unaffected (15). Certain intrauterine deformation and growth modification can, however, be sustained by the fetus after this susceptible time, as for example in the case already mentioned of hydrocephalus resulting from hypovitaminosis A late in gestation in the rabbit (27).

It is not only the developmental stage of the embryo which is important, but also the genetic constitution. For the reaction to a specific agent may vary not only between species, but also within species, between different strains or groups and even between different individuals. Genetic factors may be important at several levels. The genotype of the embryo may influence the way environmental factors are transported across the placenta or fetal membranes, and whether or not they are bound or destroyed by this barrier. This may modify the amount of an exogenous agent which actually reaches the embryo. Once in the embryo, the fetal genotype may govern the degree of binding of the substance to plasma proteins and thus the facility for transport around the body. It may influence the way the substances are concentrated in one particular tissue. It affects the way the fetal tissues metabolize and excrete the substance and thus the duration of its action. The fetal genotype also governs whether the individual has the particular determinants present necessary for its action. All these factors are important in defining whether or not an individual embryo responds to a teratogenic insult.

In a similar manner, however, the genotype of the mother will influence the teratogenic potential of an exogenous agent. Her ability to absorb and transport the substance, to bind, metabolize, store and excrete it depends upon metabolic processes and their enzyme systems which are largely genetically determined. Her overall physiological state together with any co-existing pathological condition will influence the amount and form of an environmental agent as it is presented to the fetus.

Therefore, it is important to remember that the developing embryo cannot be considered in isolation, for it is only part of an inter-related whole. The conceptus is inextricably bound to its mother, and together they form a complex interacting system. It is for this reason that *in vitro* studies, though giving valuable information on specific abnormal developmental mechanisms are of limited value in trying to elucidate the whole situation, and *in vivo* studies are of complimentary importance. Although many agents act directly on the fetus, there are some which act indirectly by, for example, reducing overall placental transfer or modifying fetal nutrition, or even more indirectly by altering maternal metabolism. Nutritional factors, especially vitamins and their co-factors are essential to many enzymatic activities involved in normal metabolic processes of the cells of both mother and fetus. A deficiency of one or several of these factors would impair these vital pathways, and while this is likely to be more devastating to the rapidly proliferating and differentiating cells of the embryo, the effects elsewhere and their sequelae cannot be discounted.

With this background in mind, observations on an animal model for NTD, the curly-tail mouse, and findings in its response to an administered exogenous agent, vitamin A, are described and related to the situation in humans.

The curly-tail gene (*ct*) arose spontaneously in 1950 and was put on a CBA background and described by Grüneberg in 1954 (17) (CBA is one of the conventional strains of laboratory mouse, derived by selective breeding.) The gene is recessive with partial penetrance, and around 60% of the mice have NTD. There is variable expressivity, so the mice may exhibit exencephaly, which is the rodent form of human anencephaly, lumbo-sacral spina bifida, which may or may not be lethal, and a variety of tail defects manifest as curls or kinks or coils, which arise because of delayed closure of the posterior neuropore (7, 17). Any such mice are described as "having NTD" or "being affected". Around 40% of the mice are phenotypically normal, but breeding experiments have shown that all mice, whatever their phenotype are homozygous for the curly-tail gene (12).

There is a female excess in affected mice, which is especially marked in exencephaly, and in individuals with spina bifida which survive, hydrocephalus may develop (12). Also, polyhydramnios and elevated amniotic alphafetoprotein levels occur in the conceptuses where there are open lesions (1). Thus, on a number of counts, aspects of the NTD of these mice resemble those of humans.

The influence of the genetic component in the cause of NTD can be seen in outcrossing experiments. F_1 hybrids between curly-tail mice and two unrelated strains of mice, which have a low spontaneous incidence of NTD – the A strain and the BALB/c do not have NTD. The abnormalities reappear however, when the F_1 mice are backcrossed to their curly-tail parents. The incidence of NTD in this backcross generation is less than the expected 50% if the *ct* gene were fully penetrant, showing that other genes in the genome are affecting its manifestation. Further, the actual incidence differs according to the strain involved in the outcross, and the difference is statistically significant. NTD occur in 24% of offspring with the BALB/c mice and in 8% with the A strain (12). Thus, these two strains are providing different genetic backgrounds, which modify the expression of the curly-tail gene to different extents.

The genetic component creates the liability in the affected individual itself, the fetus is "at risk" for NTD because of the genes it, itself, possesses, irrespective of the maternal genotype. This is shown by transplanting curly-tail embryos at the blastocyst stage, for completion of development, to the uterus of a pseudopregnant foster mother of the A strain – a non-genetically predisposed strain. NTD occurred in the embryos, and there was no significant difference in the incidence in these embryos compared with controls which had been transplanted to curly-tail recipients (33).

Further, NTDs arise in curly-tail embryos in the total absence of the maternal genotype. Mouse embryos can be cultured *in vitro* from the early headfold stage, through the period of neurulation. Non-mutant mice success-fully closed both neuropores under such conditions, but around 60% of curly-tail embryos failed to do so (7).

Vitamin A, as mentioned previously, is teratogenic to the rodent CNS, and genetic differences in susceptibility to this teratogen can be demon-strated when it is administered simultaneously to pregnant curly-tail and A strain mice. Various doses were given intraperitoneally as retinoic acid in arachis oil on day 8 of pregnancy (day of plug = day 0). The embryos were removed and examined on day 16. In the curly-tail mice, with only 5 mg/kg vitamin A, the number of NTDs in the embryos was increased. With increasing doses, the number of affected embryos rose, and by 40 mg/kg all surviving mice had NTD. In the A strain, on the other hand, these same doses had very little effect. There were no NTDs with 5, 10 and 15 mg/kg, and with 40 mg/kg only 3% of the mice had NTD. Even when 100 mg/kg was used, a dose which was lethal to curly-tail embryos, only 66% of A strain mice had NTD (34). The curly-tail mice were thus much more susceptible to the teratogen than the A strain.

Within the curly-tail mice however, with the lower doses of vitamin A, not all mice developed NTD. Five and 10 mg/kg produced NTD in around 70% (that is around 10% above the background incidence produced by the gene alone) and 15 and 20 mg/kg resulted in around 75% with NTD. Thus within a genetically predisposed strain, some mice responded to vitamin A and some did not. Within one strain, genetic differences operated rendering some individuals susceptible and some not, although this could also be accounted for by environmental differences.

These experiments also demonstrate a clear gene-environment interaction in the cause of NTD, proof that the postulated triggering effect of an environmental agent on genetically predisposed individuals can produce NTD.

The response to NTD-inducing exogenous agents is very specific, how-ever, for curly-tail mice are not susceptible to another well-known teratogen of the rodent CNS, trypan blue. A dose known to be effective in certain other mouse strains produced no increase in NTD in the curly-tail mice (32).

While their response to yet another CNS teratogen, hydroxyurea, was no overall increase in incidence of NTD, but an increase in anterior neuropore and decrease in posterior neuropore defects (36).

The genetic factors which determine the response to an environmental agent are not restricted to either the maternal or the fetal compartments but are manifested independently in both. As previously mentioned, F_1 hybrids between A strain and curly-tail mice do not have NTD. But, NTD can be induced in them by maternal administration of vitamin A on day 8 of pregnancy. In the pure parental crosses, with 40 mg/kg, 100% of curly-tail embryos (from ct female × ct male matings) have NTD, while only 3% of A embryos (A female × A male) have NTD. The F_1 hybrids have incidences of NTD intermediate between these, but the actual incidence depends on whether the F_1 hybrid has been derived from a cross between a curly-tail female and an A strain male (78%) or an A strain female and a curly-tail male (49%). The incidence is consistently and significantly higher if the curly-tail is the mother (37). In both cases, the genetic constitution of the embryo is the same, and the exogenous agent is the same, the only difference is the maternal genotype. Presumably it is exerting its effect on how vitamin A is being bound or transported, stored or metabolized by the mother, and consequently, in what proportion and in what way it reaches the fetal compartment (31).

In addition, however, these experiments show that the fetal genotype, quite separately from the maternal, also affects the response to the environmental agent. When comparing the A female × A male mating, and the A female × ct male cross, the incidences of NTD in the embryos following maternal administration of vitamin A are 3% and 49% respectively – a marked difference. In this instance, the maternal genotypes are the same, but the fetal genotypes are different. Thus the genetic constitution of the fetus is governing the differential response to vitamin A.

How very critical the timing of exposure to the environmental agent in organogenesis is in influencing the outcome, can be seen when the effects are compared of the same dose of vitamin A (5 mg/kg), given on any one day, from days 7 to 10 of pregnancy of the curly-tail mouse (Table 2). When administered on day 7 there was no alteration in the incidence of NTD in the offspring. When given on day 8, as previously described, the number of NTDs was increased. But when given on days 9 and 10, the incidences of NTDs were actually decreased, below that spontaneously occurring (normally around 60%) to 28% and 48% respectively (34). This phenomenon is especially significant with treatment on day 9.

This is a paradoxical situation where the same amount of the same substance has two opposite effects at different times in embryogenesis. Of special importance is the finding that in mice with a genetic predisposition to

Table 2. The effect of maternal administration of a single dose of 5 mg/kg vitamin A as retinoic acid in arachis oil on different days of gestation in the curly-tail mouse.

	Controls (Arachis oil alone)	Vitamin A			
		day 7	day 8	day 9	day 10
Total live fetuses	113	55	34	204	62
Number of fetuses with NTD (%)	65 (58)	32 (58)	24 (71)	58 (28)	30 (48)

NTD, under certain circumstances, the maternal administration of a nutritional factor can actually prevent NTD occurring. This seems to parallel findings in the multivitamin prevention study in humans.

The somewhat bizarre finding that vitamin A exerts a teratogenic effect when administered to the mother on day 8 and a curative effect when given on day 9 perhaps needs some explanation if it is to be accepted as plausible. The probable key to the issue lies in the relative speed with which embryogenesis takes place in the mouse. What takes a week in man, takes little more than a day in the mouse. With regard to formation of the neural tube, on day 8 in the mouse, the embryo, little more than a flattened plate of three layers of cells, elongates, the midline neural groove deepens, the neural folds rise up and fusion occurs first in the lower cervical region, then concurrently both anteriorly and posteriorly from this point (Figure 1). On day 9 (Figure 2), the neural tube is largely formed, and what essentially remains to be achieved is the closure of the two neuropores. It is possible that these two events in neurulation, as observed on day 8 and day 9, involve different mechanisms, which are influenced in different ways by vitamin A (31a). Evidence that this might be so comes from high power scanning electron microscope studies. On day 8, in untreated mice, along the crest of the contralateral neural folds close to the fusion site there is a line of cells on which there are a number of compact cell membrane processes (lamellipodia) and some longer membranous processes. In vitamin A treated mice, the density and number of these processes is markedly increased. There is thus an observable difference between normal and vitamin A treated mice. On day 9 on the other hand, when the neuropores are closing, the appearance between the two types of mice is similar. In both there is a continuous line of dense lamellipodia all around the neuropore. It is thus possible to suggest that on day 8, vitamin A prevents closure of the neural tube (its teratogenic effect) by increasing the number of membranous processes above normal,

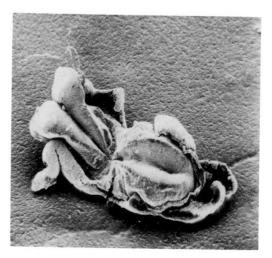

Fig. 1. Scanning electron microscope picture of an early stage in the formation of the neural tube in the mouse, day 8 of gestation (× 60).

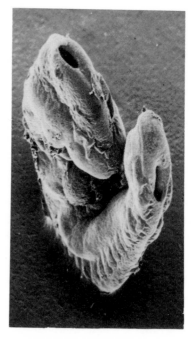

Fig. 2. Later stage, day 9 of gestation in the mouse. The neural tube is largely formed, leaving the closure of the two neuropores to be achieved (× 60).

while on day 9 an increased number of these processes is a normal part of neuropore closure, and so on this day, vitamin A enhances the natural process and so aids closure of the neural tube.

When vitamin A was used on day 8 as a teratogen, there was a dose level where all surviving embryos could be made to have NTD. However, when used as a curative agent on day 9, by contrast, there was no dose which cured all the mice. With different dose levels there was a V-shaped response, 5 mg/kg had the maximum effect, 1, 10 and 20 mg/kg had lesser, though still significant curative effects (35). Thus, not only is the timing of the curative agent important, but also the actual dose, there is one dose which is of optimum benefit. However, even if both these criteria are met, not all individuals are cured.

Analogies between these experiments in the curly-tail mouse and the human vitamin supplementation programme lead to speculation as to whether vitamin A could be teratogenic in man or whether it could be the effective agent. Both are thought unlikely, because the mouse experiments involve doses of vitamin A of a vastly different order from that being administered to the women. The teratogenic doses in the curly-tail mice are 10–40 mg/kg, which is 33 000–133 000 IU/kg. The curative day 9 dose is 16 000 IU/kg. The daily dose of vitamin A which the women receive in Pregnavite forte F is 4000 IU which represents approximately 70 IU/kg (35).

Finally, Pregnavite forte F, at a dose roughly equivalent to twice the human daily dose, has been administered by stomach tube continuously pre- and post-conceptionally to the curly-tail mice, and as a single dose specifically on day 7 or day 8 of pregnancy. In other experiments, a variety of doses of folic acid, or folinic acid, or vitamin B_{12} have been administered to pregnant curly-tail mice on different gestational days. None of these regimes had any effect on the incidence of NTD in the offspring (31, 32 and unpublished data).

Extrapolation of any animal experiment to man is fraught with uncertainty. It would seem reasonable to assume that the final prevention of human NTD will only be effected by studies in Man. Nevertheless animals are not without value, and animal studies have provided some useful insights into the cause and prevention of NTD by maternal nutritional factors.

Acknowledgements

Experimental work in the curly-tail mouse has been performed with the generous financial assistance of Action Research – The National Fund for Research into Crippling Diseases, which is gratefully acknowledged.

References

1. Adinolfi, M., Beck, S., Embury, S., Polani, P. E. and Seller, M. J. (1976). Levels of α-fetoprotein in amniotic fluids of mice (curly-tail) with neural tube defects. *J. Med. Genetics* **13**, 511–513.
2. Baranov, V. S. (1966). The specificity of the teratogenic effect of aminopterin as compared to other teratogenic agents. *Bull. Exp. Biol.* (Russian) **1**, 77–82.
3. Bernhardt, I. B. and Dorsey, D. J. (1974). Hypervitaminosis A and congenital renal anomalies in the human infant. *Obstet. Gynaecol.* **43**, 750–755.
4. Carter, C. O. (1974). Clues to the aetiology of neural tube malformations. *Devel. Med. Child Neurol.* **16**, Supplement 32, 3–15.
5. Cheng, D. W., Bairnson, T. A., Rao, A. N. and Subbammal, S. (1960). Effect of variations of rations on the incidence of teratogeny in vitamin E deficient rats. *J. Nutrition* **71**, 54–60.
6. Cohlan, S. Q. (1954). Congenital anomalies in the rat produced by the excessive intake of vitamin A during pregnancy. *Pediatrics* **13**, 556–569.
7. Copp, A. J., Seller, M. J. and Polani, P. E. (1982). Neural tube development in mutant (curly-tail) and normal mouse embryos: the timing of posterior neuropore closure *in vivo* and *in vitro*. *J. Exp. Embryol. Morphol.* **69**, 151–167.
8. Curley, F. J., Ingalls, T. H. and Zappasodi, P. (1968). 6-aminonicotinamide-induced skeletal malformations in mice. *Arch. Environ. Health* **16**, 309–315.
9. Davis, S. D., Nelson, T. and Shepard, T. H. (1970). Teratogenicity of vitamin B(6) deficiency: omphalocele skeletal and neural defects, and splenic hypoplasia. *Science* **169**, 1329–1330.
10. Dreosti, I. E., Grey, P. C. and Wilkins, P. J. (1972). Deoxyribonucleic acid synthesis, protein synthesis and teratogenesis in zinc deficient rats. *S. Afr. Med. J.* **46**, 1585–1588.
11. Duncan, J. R. and Hurley, L. S. (1978). An interaction between zinc and vitamin A in pregnant and fetal rats. *J. Nutrition* **108**, 1431–1438.
12. Embury, S., Seller, M. J., Adinolfi, M. and Polani, P. E. (1979). Neural tube defects in curly-tail mice. I. Incidence and expression. *Proc. Roy. Soc. Lond. B.* **206**, 85–94.
13. Fraser, F. C. (1980). Evolution of a palatable multifactorial threshold model. *Am. J. Human Genet.* **32**, 796–813.
14. Friedman, W. F. and Mills, L. F. (1969). The relationship between vitamin D and the craniofacial and dental anomalies of the supravalvular aortic stenosis syndrome. *Pediatrics* **43**, 12–18.
15. Giroud, A. and Martinet, M. (1956). Teratogenese par hautes doses de vitamin A en fonction des stades du developpement. *Arch. Anat. Micros. Morph. Exp.* **45**, 77–98.
16. Giroud, A. and Martinet, M. (1959). Teratogenese par hypervitaminose A chez le rat, la souris, le cobaye et le lapin. *Arch. Franç. Pédiatrie.* **16**, 1–5.
17. Grüneberg, H. (1954). Genetical studies on the skeleton of the mouse. VIII. Curly-tail. *J. Genet.* **52**, 52–67.
18. Hale, F. (1933). Pigs born without eyeballs. *J. Heredity* **24**, 105–106.
19. Hale, F. (1935). Relation of vitamin A to anophthalmos in pigs. *Am. J. Ophthal.* **18**, 1087–1093.

20. Hale, F. (1937). Relation of maternal vitamin A deficiency to microphthalmia in pigs. *Texas State J. Med.* **33**, 228–232.
21. Hook, E. B., Healy, K. M., Niles, A. M. and Skalko, R. G. (1974). Vitamin E: A teratogen or antiteratogen? *Lancet* **i**, 809.
22. Horvath, C., Szonyi, L. and Mold, K. (1976). Preventive effect of riboflavin and ATP on the teratogenic effects of the phenothiazine derivative T-28. *Teratology* **14**, 167–170.
23. Hurley, L. S. and Shrader, R. E. (1972). Congenital malformations of the nervous system in zinc deficient rats. *In* "Neuro-biology of the Trace Metals Zinc and Copper" (C. C. Pfeiffer, ed.) pp. 7–51. Academic Press, London and New York.
24. Hurley, L. S. and Swenerton, H. (1966). Congenital malformations resulting from zinc deficiency in rats. *Proc. Soc. Exp. Biol. Med.* **123**, 692–697.
25. Lefebvres-Boisselot, J. (1951). Role tératogène de la déficience en acide panthothénique chez le rat. *Ann. Médicine* **52**, 225–298.
26. Marin-Padilla, M. and Ferm, V. H. (1965). Somite necrosis and developmental malformations induced by vitamin A in the golden hamster. *J. Embryol. Exp. Morphol.* **13**, 1–8.
27. Millen, J. W., Woollam, D. H .M. and Lamming, G. E. (1953). Hydrocephalus associated with deficiency of vitamin A. *Lancet* **ii**, 1234–1236.
28. Momose, Y., Akiyoshi, S., Mori, K., Nishimura, N., Fujishima, H., Imaizumi, S. and Agata, I. (1972). On teratogenicity of vitamin E. Reports from the Department of Anatomy, Mie Perfectural University School of Medicine, **20**, 27–35.
29. Nelson, M. M., Wright, H. V., Asling, C. W., Evans, H. M. (1955). Multiple congenital abnormalities resulting from transitory deficiency of pteroylglutamic acid during gestation in the rat. *J. Nutrition* **56**, 349–370.
30. Palludan, B. (1966). Swine in teratological studies. *In* "Swine in Biomedical Research" (L. K. Bustad and R. O. McClella eds) pp. 51–78. Frayn Printing, Seattle, Washington.
31. Seller, M. J. (1981). An essay on research into the causation and prevention of spina bifida. *Zeit. Kinderchirurgie* **34**, 306–314.
31a. Seller, M. J. (1983). Neural tube defects: cause and prevention. *In* "Paediatric Research: A Genetic Approach" (M. Adinolfi, P. F. Benson, F. Giannelli, M. J. Seller eds) Spastics International Medical Publications, London.
32. Seller, M. J. and Adinolfi, M. (1981). The curly-tail mouse: An experimental model for human neural tube defects. *Life Sciences* **29**, 1607–1615.
33. Seller, M. J., Beck, S. E., Adinolfi, M. and Polani, P. E. (1981). Maternal environment and the expression of murine neural tube defects. *Prenatal Diagnosis* **1**, 103–105.
34. Seller, M. J., Embury, S., Polani, P. E. and Adinolfi, M. (1979). Neural tube defects in curly-tail mice. II. Effect of maternal administration of vitamin A. *Proc. Roy. Soc. London B.* **206**, 95–107.
35. Seller, M. J. and Perkins, K. J. (1982). Prevention of neural tube defects in curly-tail mice by maternal administration of vitamin A. *Prenatal Diagnosis* **2**, 297–300.
36. Seller, M. J. and Perkins, K. J. (1982). Effect of hydroxyurea on neural tube defects in the curly-tail mouse. *J. Craniofacial Genet. Develop. Biol* (in press).
37. Seller, M. J., Perkins, K. J. and Adinolfi, M. (1982). Differential response of

heterozygous curly-tail mouse embryos to vitamin A teratogenesis depending on maternal genotype. *Teratology* (in press).
38. Skalko, R. G. and Gold, M. P. (1974). Teratogenicity of methotrexate in mice. *Teratology* **9**, 159–164.
39. Smithells, R. W., Sheppard, S. and Schorah, C. J. (1976). Vitamin deficiencies and neural tube defects. *Arch. Dis. Child.* **51**, 944–950.
40. Smithells, R. W., Sheppard, S., Schorah, C. J., Seller, M. J., Nevin, N. C., Harris, R., Read, A. P. and Fielding, D. W. (1980). Possible prevention of neural tube defects by periconceptional vitamin supplementation. *Lancet* **i**, 339–340.
41. Smithells, R. W., Sheppard, S., Schorah, C. J., Seller, M. J., Nevin, N. C., Harris, R., Read, A. P. and Fielding, D. W. (1981). Apparent prevention of neural tube defects by periconceptional vitamin supplementation. *Arch. Dis. Child.* **56**, 911–918.
42. Smithells, R. W., Sheppard, S., Schorah, C. J., Seller, M. J., Nevin, N. C., Harris, R., Read, A. P., Fielding, D. W. and Walker, S. (1981). Vitamin supplementation and neural tube defects. *Lancet* **ii**, 1425.
43. Tuchmann-Duplessis, H., Lefebvres-Boisselot, J. and Mercier-Parot, L. (1959). L'action tératogène de l'acide x-methyl-folique sur diverses éspeces animales. *Arch. Franç. Pédiatrie* **15**, 509–520.
44. Warkany, J. (1943). Effect of maternal rachitogenic diet on skeletal development of young rat. *Am. J. Dis. Child.* **66**, 511–516.
45. Warkany, J. and Kalter, H. (1959). Experimental production of congenital malformations in mammals by metabolic procedure. *Physiol. Rev.* **39**, 69–115.
46. Warkany, J. and Petering, H. G. (1972). Congenital malformations of the central nervous system in rats produced by maternal zinc deficiency. *Teratology* **5**, 319–334.
47. Warkany, J. and Schraffenberger, E. (1944). Congenital malformations of the eyes induced in rats by maternal vitamin A deficiency. *Proc. Soc. Exp. Biol. Med.* **57**, 49–52.
48. Wilson, J. G. and Warkany, J. (1948). Malformations in the genito-urinary tract induced by maternal vitamin A deficiency in the rat. *Am. J. Anat.* **83**, 357–407.
49. Wilson, J. G. and Warkany, J. (1950). Cardiac and aortic arch anomalies in the offspring of vitamin A deficient rats correlated with similar human anomalies. *Pediatrics* **5**, 708–725.
50. Woodard, J. C. and Newberne, P. M. (1966). Relation of vitamin B_{12} and one-carbon metabolism to hydrocephalus in the rat. *J. Nutrition* **88**, 375–381.

Commentary

Felix Beck: I would take issue with the statement that ". . . the embryo is only vulnerable to environmental assault for a relatively short time in its prenatal life". Whilst agreeing that the pre-gastrulation embryo is effectively unresponsive to teratogenic agents it is now clear that, although many of the major anatomical defects are caused by disturbances of morphogenesis during the embryonic period, dramatic effects are nevertheless caused by a variety of agents acting during the fetal and even the early post-natal period. Cases of microcephaly have undoubtedly been associated with the atomic explosions in Hiroshima and Nagasaki and both ionization radiations as well as nutritional deficiencies have been shown to affect growth and the establishment of normal cerebral function when the conceptus is exposed to them at the very end of the gestation period. Nutritional lack may also result from placental insufficiency.

The statement is made that:

> Once in the embryo the fetal genotype may govern the degree of binding of the substance to plasma proteins and thus the facility for transport around the body. It may influence the way the substances are concentrated in one particular tissue. It affects the way the fetal tissues metabolise and excrete the substance and thus the duration of its action. The fetal genotype also governs whether the individual has the particular determinants present necessary for its action. All these factors are important in defining whether or not an individual embryo responds to a teratogenic insult.

Whilst in general agreement with this point of view insofar as it is of importance during late embryonic and fetal life, it does seem likely that genotypic differences between mammalian species are less marked during early embryonic existence – particularly before the establishment of a fully functional fetal heart and a chorio-allantoic placenta. Clearly this is a very general statement but it is in keeping with the theory of recapitulation and can, to some extent, be supported by the demonstration of Shepard and his group (2) to the effect that early embryonic energy production depends upon glycolysis and the pentosephosphate shunt; the Krebs cycle having not yet been activated.

Because early mammalian embryos have more in common than they do in the later fetal stages there is much to be said for *in vitro* studies. *In vitro* whole embryo cultures can be carried out on embryos lying within the extra-embryonic membranes between the primitive streak stage and the early limb bud state (i.e. to a stage at which the neural tube has fully closed). The fact that such a culture deals only with the embryo and its membranes and leaves out any maternal effect is both a strength and a weakness. Its strength lies in the fact that factors acting directly on the embryo can be precisely analysed. The weakness – the fact that maternal metabolism is not involved can, to a large extent, be overcome by administering the putative teratogen to an adult animal and using the serum from that animal for the subsequent culture. This is particularly well shown in the case of chlorambucil which is ineffective when placed directly into the culture medium but highly teratogenic when an embryo is cultured in the serum from a chlorambucil-treated mother. With the development of culture in human serum it becomes possible to approach the investigation of a teratogenic situation in man by relatively direct means. Whilst not suggesting that such a method should replace *in vivo* testing it does have certain advantages which enable it to be extrapolated in a situation where a difference exists between the adult metabolism of man and the rat or mouse.

The curly-tailed mouse is an interesting model for neural tube defect in man but the fact that there is a female excess in affected mice in late gestation does not necessarily indicate that its pathogenesis is particularly closely related to the human condition although, indeed, the possibility is a very real one. One would expect hydrocephalus, polyhydramnios and elevated amniotic alpha-protein levels in conceptuses where there are open lesions to occur with any type of spina bifida.

It is true that ". . . the maternal administration of a nutritional factor can actually prevent neural tube defects from occurring" at certain stages of its development in the curly-tailed mouse. The parallel between this situation in which a nutritional factor (vitamin A) overcomes a predominantly genetic condition does not seem to me to be closely parallel to the recent work on vitamin supplementation in "at risk" women because in the latter the risk is probably due to a predominantly environmentally conditioned circumstance namely that of relative vitamin deficiency. As always one has to bear in mind that in all biological situations both genetic and environmental factors play some part.

I am particularly interested in the fact that curly-tailed mice do not show particular susceptibility to other teratogens causing neural tube defects such as trypan blue. This once again underlines the likelihood that numerous factors might cause non-closure of the neural tube and that not all of these may be operative in every situation. Indeed, it makes the analogy betwen the basic pathogenesis of the neural tube defect in curly-tailed mice and that in human vitamin-deficient states a tenuous one.

Trypan blue does not specifically produce NTD. It works by inhibiting pinocytosis in the extraembryonic membranes (3). The compound as bought commercially is notoriously impure (1) and results obtained from impurified samples are virtually valueless.

It is possible on morphological grounds that the anterior or posterior neuropores close by different mechanisms to those prevailing in the rest of the neural tube.

1. Beck, F. and Lloyd, J. B. (1966). *In* "Advances in Teratology" (D. H. M. Woolham, ed.) Vol. 1. Lagos Press.
2. Shepard, T. H., Tanimura, T. and Robkin, M. (1970). Energy metabolism in early mammalian embryos. *Dev. Biol.* Suppl. **4**, 42–58.
3. Williams, K. E., Roberts, G., Kidston, E. M., Beck, F. and Lloyd, J. B. (1976). Inhibition of pinocytosis in the rat yolk sac by trypan blue. *Teratology* **14**, 343–354.

Norman Nevin: This is an excellent, in depth, appraisal of the state of the art of the teratogenic effect of nutritional deficiencies in experimental animals. Her work with the curly tail mice and vitamin A shows clearly the importance of both the genetic and the environmental components in the aetiology of NTDs. There is always the difficulty in extrapolating from animal experiments to man, but the model she has developed will help in the understanding of the pathogenesis of the lesions in NTDs.

The statement ". . . in some cases deficiencies of certain vitamins may interact with deficiencies with other substances . . ." (p. 3) is important. There are several examples where vitamins may ameliorate the teratogenic effect of an agent. It is possible that vitamin C may be important in ameliorating the teratogenic effect of folic acid deficiency. Laurence and colleagues have shown a definite association of poor maternal diet with NTDs, pointing towards a more generalised than a single deficiency.

Michael Laurence: This is a succinct account of the diverse effects of the various vitamin deficiencies and excesses on different species of experimental animal. In particular it refers to the causation of NTD by excessive doses of vitamin A in the mouse, guinea pig, rabbit, hamster and pig.

Although it is true in general that "the embryo is only vulnerable to environmental assault for a relatively short time in its prenatal life", intrauterine damage later in the pregnancy can give rise to malformations. Examples are hypovitaminosis A in the rabbit, giving rise to congenital hydrocephalus and certain infections such as with cytomegalic inclusion disease virus causing hydrocephalus and eye abnormalities in man, and also amniotic bands in man giving rise to intrauterine amputation.

Seller illustrates well the way the maternal and the fetal genotype separately can influence the way a particular teratogen might affect the embryonic development and how complex and bound up the fetal maternal axis is. However, the curly tailed mouse seems to be homozygous for its susceptibility to neural tube defect, but even here there is variable expressivity, presumably due to multifactorial and possibly polygenic factors. The actual experiments involving the curly-tailed mouse quoted in this paper cannot, I think, be faulted, but they cannot be applied directly to the causation of neural tube defects in man.

Although there are few instances where a woman has taken vast amounts of vitamin A during pregnancy and fewer reports where this has led to malformation, let alone neural tube defect, it is conceivable that under certain circumstances a dangerous dose of vitamin A might be consumed by a woman taking multivitamin preparations, as may have happened in one of our patients that should have been supplemented by pre-conceptional folic acid. A woman who might realize that she has become pregnant earlier than planned and not supplemented as planned, may in an attempt to make up for the lack of supplementation at the right moment be panicked into swallowing large quantities of tablets at once. It would take only just over 200 tablets to reach the dose in a 70 kg woman equivalent to that which caused an increase in the incidence of neural tube defects in the curly-tailed mouse.

John Edwards: The word periconceptional is unfortunate. The evidence is of supplementation before the development of the lesion, known to be 2–3 weeks after conception. There is no evidence that the supplementation before conception helps. Small molecules like folic acid would be expected to reach equilibrium levels in a few days.

The concept of multifactorial with triggers is, I think, so obvious, and so well described in the vernacular by many authors, especially Hippocrates, that it should not appear in its polysyllabic finery in scientific discussions. The confusion generated by this elaboration of the obvious has done more than anything else to divert teratologists from the orderly and direct search for teratogens.

I think this is a most valuable and solid survey, which places the problem in context, and disposes of the myth of vitamin A teratogenicity at physiological levels.

The author is a little hard on the pre-thalidomide workers. The key papers of Record and McKeown on CNS malformations preceded thalidomide, as did the paper from Aberdeen.

1. Edwards, J. H. (1958). Malformations of the central nervous system in Scotland. *Brit. J. Prev. Soc. Med.* **12**, 115.
2. McKeown, T. and Record, R. G. (1951). Seasonal incidence of congenital malformations of the central nervous system. *Lancet* **i**, 192.
3. MacMahon, B., Puch, T. F. and Ingalls, T. H. (1953). Anencephalus, spina bifida and hydrocephalus. Incidence related to sex, race, and season of birth, and incidence in siblings. *Brit. J. Prev. Soc. Med.* **7**, 211.
4. Record, R. G. and McKeown, T. (1950). Congenital malformations of the central nervous system. II. Maternal reproductive history and familial incidence. *Brit. J. Prev. Soc. Med.* **4**, 26.

Chris Schorer: The paper by Seller shows clearly how the genetic and environmental components of NTD are closely linked, the influence of environmental factors being affected by the genetic predisposition of both the mother and the fetus. The timing of the environmental insult is also shown to be critical and different for different malformations.

Whilst supporting an environmental factor in the causation of NTD, these studies show the difficulty of extrapolating animal findings to man because of the way the genotype of the animal can influence its susceptibility to the environment. Differences in this susceptibility from species to species suggest that we should not be discouraged that the vitamins associated with NTD in human studies, such as folic acid, have not been shown to be effective in reducing the incidence in the curly-tail mouse. It is, however, worth emphasizing that as far as I am aware there are no studies using whole animals which have succeeded in increasing the prevalence of NTD by maternal dietary restriction of folic acid alone. There is a report showing a decrease in the incidence of hydrocephalus in the rat when the dams were given folic acid (2), but an increased frequency of NTD has only been reported when folate antagonists and/or antibiotics have been included in the dietary regime (Chapter 1) (1). There have been few animal studies which have investigated the affect of combined deficiencies of a number of micronutrients and there is evidence that these may be more damaging to the developing fetus than the restriction of a single nutrient (unpublished work).

The failure of folic acid supplementation to reduce the incidence of NTD in the curly tail mouse could be explained in many ways. It may not be involved in the aetiology of NTD in this species. The limiting process could be the failure of appropriate cellular interactions occurring in the developmental process at the time of closure of the neural tube and a reduced rate of cell division, which would be encouraged by depletion of folic acid, may have no part to play in causation of NTD in this species. The one nutrient found to affect the incidence of NTD in these mice is vitamin A. Apart from its role in the visual process the function of this vitamin is not understood, but it would be interesting to speculate on a possible role in maintaining appropriate cellular interactions. If the rate of cell division is not the critical factor in this species, folate antagonists, which increase the prevalence of NTD in other species (1), presumably by disrupting the process of cell division, would have little effect on the incidence of NTD in the curly tail mouse, provided that the rate of cell division did not become the limiting factor in the closure of the neural tube.

1. Nelson, M. M. (1960). Teratogenic effects of P.G.A. deficiency in the rat. *In* "Congenital Malformations", (G. E. W. Wolstenholme and C. M. O'Connell, eds) p. 134. Ciba Foundation Symposium, Churchill, London.
2. O'Dell, B. L., Whitley, J. R. and Hogan, A. C. (1948). Relation of folic acid and vitamin A to incidence of hydrocephalus in the infant rat. *Proc. Soc. Expt. Biol. Med.* **69**, 272.

D. Kirke: The great advantage of animals in scientific research is, as Seller points out, that they can be manipulated in ways in which humans cannot. Although fully aware of the difficulties of extrapolating findings from animal studies to man, I would like to make two points about the relevance of animal studies to the current work on vitamin supplementation in the prevention of neural tube defects in man.

If periconceptional vitamin supplementation is shown by randomized control trials to be effective in reducing the risk of recurrence of neural tube defect, then it is likely that vitamin supplementation regimes in use in the population would be of the same duration as those employed by Smithells and his colleagues (1) and in the randomized trials. However, supplementation of approximately 10 weeks' duration, as recommended in the Smithells study (1), may be unnecessary. It may be that supplementation for several days around the time of neural tube closure may achieve the same result as supplementation for two months. It would be difficult to test this experimentally in humans, particularly if randomized trials should confirm the efficacy of vitamin supplementation using the same duration of supplementation as Smithells *et al.* (1). Animal studies of the critical time period for supplementation such as that described by Seller *et al.* (2) would shed light on this.

Such work would be important for two practical reasons. Firstly, with regard to the primary prevention of neural tube defects, most mothers are some 14–21 days post-conception before they suspect or know that they are pregnant. As the neural tube closes at about 22–26 days after conception, it might be that supplementation from the date of suspicion of pregnancy would be effective. In the event of randomized trials confirming the efficacy and safety of vitamin supplementation, there would be little to be lost in supplementing such mothers post-conceptionally but the results of these trials will not be available for several years. In the meantime one would like to see support for such a policy from animal studies. Secondly, there is the obvious financial advantage of shorter term supplementation.

1. Smithells, R. W., Sheppard, S., Schorah, C. J., Seller, M. J., Nevin, N. C., Harris, R., Read, A. P., Fielding, D. W. (1981). Apparent prevention of neural tube defects by periconceptional vitamin supplementation. *Arch. Dis. Child.* **56**, 911–918.
2. Seller, M. J., Embury, S., Polani, P. E. and Adinolfi, M. (1979). Neural tube defects in curly-tail mice. II. Effect of maternal administration of vitamin A. *Proc. Roy. Soc. Lond. B.* **206**, 95–107.

Nicholas Wald: It would be helpful if the data on vitamin A administration from days 7–10 of pregnancy in the curly-tailed mouse could be summarized in a table (see pp. 8 and 9). How plausible is it to have a teratogenic effect on one day and a curative effect on the next? It is said that Pregnavite forte F administration to curly-tailed mice does not reduce the risk of neural tube defects. Can the data be given? How do these negative results affect our interpretation of the human results?

Editor's note: See also Appendix III.

Ian Leck: This clearly written review of mainly *in vivo* studies of teratogenic effects of vitamin deficiencies and excesses in rodents, and Beck's account of the potentialities of *in vitro* methods for studying these effects, seem to me to complement each other very successfully. That Seller should tend to concentrate more on the results of teratogenic experiments, and Beck (Chapter 2) more on potentialities, is of course inevitable given that *in vivo* studies, having been going on for longer and on a larger scale than mammalian studies *in vitro*, have had much more opportunity to yield results. Seller agrees that "*in vivo* studies are of complimentary importance" to *in vitro* ones. *In vivo* studies encompass changes produced or undergone by teratogens in the mother as well as in the embryo. However, having demonstrated *in vivo* that a substance is a teratogen, it is just as important to locate and identify the changes through which its teratogenic effects are mediated, and therefore to use methods such as *in vitro* culture which enable different parts of the mother–embryo complex to be considered in isolation. From the findings quoted by Beck from studies comparing embryos cultured in sera from mothers who had received a teratogen and in sera to which the same teratogen had been added directly, it seems that changes in the mother as well as changes in the embryo can sometimes be elucidated *in vitro*.

An allied need is to distinguish between the effects that the genotypes of the mother and the embryo can have on development. Seller's paper provides examples of three approaches to this problem: blastocyst transplantation, *in vitro* culture, and reciprocal crossing between animals from strains with high and low risks of neural tube defects. The incidence of neural tube defects in mice homozygous for the *ct* gene was apparently unaffected by being cultured as embryos *in vitro* or transplanted as blastocysts to mothers of strains in which neural tube defects are rare. The frequency with which maternal hypervitaminosis A led to the occurrence of neural tube defects in the offspring of matings between *ct* homozygotes and animals of a low risk-strain, on the other hand, was higher when the mother was the *ct* homozygote than when the father was. This is a surprising combination of findings, suggesting that maternal *ct* homozygosity increases the risk of

neural tube defect that heterozygous embryos face in the presence of maternal hypervitaminosis A, but does not affect the comparably high risk that
homozygous embryos face in the absence of this teratogen. It would be
interesting to see whether these conclusions could be confirmed by other
methods: for example, the risks experienced without vitamin A supplementation by the offspring of *ct* homozygous mothers and *ct* heterozygous
fathers could be compared with those for the reciprocal cross, and the risks
to *ct* heterozygote embryos could be explored after culture in sera from
females of the two parent strains who had received excess vitamin A, or after
transplantation to the uteri of such females.

The Use of Whole Embryo Culture of The Rat in the Experimental Study of Human Birth Defects

FELIX BECK

Medical School,
University of Leicester

Introduction

In the first half of this century, following the "rediscovery" of Mendel's works, birth defects were largely ascribed to genetic causes. The assumption was made that the intra-uterine environment was unassailable and little distinction was made between terms such as "congenital defects" and "genetic defects". The first clear indication that embryonic development could be perverted by environmental circumstances came over 40 years ago and, interestingly, in the particular field to which this Symposium is addressed. Warkany and his co-workers (30–32) showed that dietary deficiency in rats could cause predictable types and levels of malformation among the offspring. Invoking perhaps the most misquoted phrase in the language this work engendered little interest because "The proper study of mankind is Man". *

* The phrase "the proper study of mankind is man" comes from Pope's *Essay on Man*. Taken in context it reads: "Know then thyself, presume not God to scan, The proper study of mankind is man." and goes on to describe man as: "Great Lord of all things, yet a prey to all; Sole judge of truth, in endless errors hurled; The glory, jest and riddle of the world!" (Ep. ii 1, i.) Clearly it was not in the poet's mind to direct man's thoughts exclusively to his own anatomy. The work is at a somewhat higher plane – a sort of attempt to do the same for philosophy as Galileo and Darwin did for the physical and biological sciences. I cannot think that it is relevant to animal testing in toxicology.

Gregg's (10) discovery of the connection between maternal rubella and birth malformation produced more interest but the demonstration that the effects were due to fetal infection put them into the same category as syphilis and toxoplasmosis which were already well recognized and, to some extent, understood. It was of little surprise to those actively working in the field that in 1961 both Lenz and McBride (18, 20) described the association between thalidomide and birth defects. The general clinician was, however, quite unprepared for the event and to some extent an over-reaction occurred, with the result that almost every drug, dietary constituent or environmental pollutant has come under often quite unwarranted suspicion. Gradually a saner attitude has appeared and medical scientists are now turning back to re-examine some of the hard experimental data of the past in the context of the human situation.

After years of clinical research into neural tube defects involving many workers and giving rise to numerous false leads Smithells *et al.* (29), in a paper which expanded an earlier letter to the *Lancet* (28) produced evidence that periconceptional administration of Pregnavite forte F ® (Bencard) greatly lessened the incidence of recurrence in women who had given birth to a previous baby with NTD. The polyvitamin mixture used contains vitamins A and D, thiamine, riboflavin, pyridoxine, nicotinamide, ascorbic acid, folic acid and some minerals (see Table 1, Chapter 1) so that even if the results of this study are completely confirmed the situation will remain complex. Laurence *et al.* (16) announced work which suggested that dietary counselling before another pregnancy lessened the likelihood of a second neural tube defect occurring in the offspring. In another study Laurence *et al.* (17) suggested that folic acid was the most important of the vitamins to be considered in connection with neural tube defects in man. If this is proven it is clearly of importance in connection with the findings of Smithells *et al.* (28).

Bearing in mind all the accrued clinical evidence it is important to re-emphasize that in certain closely studied animal experiments birth defects such as cleft palate are multifactorial in origin with a polygenic background and it seems to me unlikely, therefore, that attention to diet alone – and perhaps more so to a single factor in the diet – will eliminate NTD in man completely. Furthermore, no suggestion is made by any of the workers concerned that dietary deficiencies are specifically concerned with neural tube defect. The concept of optimal critical times during gestation for the pathogenesis of various specific congenital defects has been well documented experimentally (35) as well as by the thalidomide episode (19). There is reason to believe, therefore, that if nutritional defects are a factor causing neural tube abnormalities when active early in gestation, they may equally well help to produce other malformations at later periods. Indeed,

Warkany and Nelson (30) in their first paper on the subject described the skeletal abnormalities in the offspring of rats reared on a deficient diet.

Before passing to *in vitro* techniques it is necessary to spend a moment in examining the value of *in vivo* animal experiments in the evaluation of human teratological risk. The obvious difficulties inherent in extrapolating toxicological and metabolic results from animals to man have brought animal experiments into such disrepute that many consider them to be virtually valueless or, even worse, a ritual performed by drug houses in order to satisfy appropriate licensing agencies. This is emphatically not the case. By and large animal experiments allow us to say that under stipulated conditions the probability of untoward effects resulting from a certain environmental insult to human populations will be low. Palmer (25) and many before him have contributed to the development of logical techniques of assessing the risks incurred from drugs and other environmental insults which latter would include dietary defects. For example, among many factors, they have paid attention to matters such as the level and duration of action of a noxious stimulus and its relationship to changes in the maternal plasma (e.g. in concentrations of a drug) as well as changing embryonic sensitivity with gestation period. The choice of parental test animal is realized to be of considerable importance not only because of its specific metabolism but also because of its placental and "preplacental" nutritional arrangements and this is taken into account in all reliable studies. Far from rapidly becoming an anachronism, whole animal teratogenic studies are likely to continue to enhance our knowledge of teratogenic processes in a variety of fields including that concerning the effects of maternal nutritional failure during pregnancy.

Quite recently New's pioneering work on the culture of vertebrate embryos has developed to a point where it has become possible to culture essentially normal rat embryos from the primitive streak or early head fold stage to the limb bud stage. The period of culture is 48 h at the end of which time the embryos have some 25–30 somites and the neural tube is closed (Figs 1 and 2). The subject is well reviewed by New (23). The development of this system marks a major milestone in research into congenital malformations and some of its multiple applications are the major subject of this contribution.

In Vitro Embryo Culture

Figure 3 is a diagram of the normal development of the rat embryo and Fig. 4 shows the way in which the embryo (in this case corresponding to 4e in Fig. 3) relies upon a transudate of rat serum to provide for its nutritional

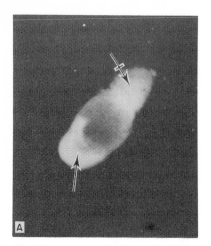
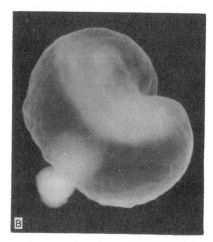

Fig. 1. (a) Nine and a half day rat conceptus prepared for explantation into culture serum (compare with Fig. 3d). The early head fold embryo is marked (↑) and the ectoplacental cone (⚓) × 12. (b) Rat embryo contained within yolk sac at 11.5 days following 48 hours of culture in rat serum (compare with Fig. 3f) × 12.

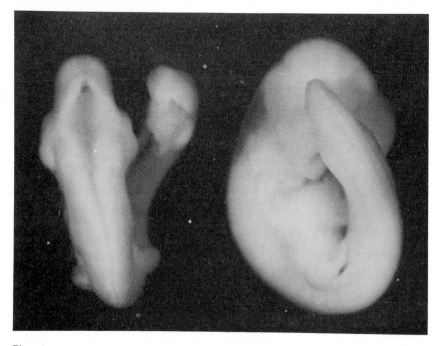

Fig. 2. Rat embryo removed from yolk sac after explantation at 9·5 days and cultured for 48 h in rat serum. × 15.

requirements. Most of the serum biopolymers endocytized by the visceral layer of the yolk sac epithelium are broken down intracellularly to provide the embryo with its nutritional needs (8) and this is illustrated in Fig. 5. The usual culture period extends from stage 3d to 3f and ends at the point at which histiotrophic nutrition is superseded by haemotrophic nutrition (see below for a discussion of these terms). The rat is particularly convenient for *in vitro* whole embryo culture because the relationship of the extra-embryonic membrane to their sources of nutrition are identical to those pertaining *in vivo*. In our own experiments the culture technique described by New *et al.* (24) was used throughout and we first validated the system by extensive morphometric measurements which showed that the levels of endocytosis *in vitro* corresponded to those calculated *in vivo* (Table 1) (11). As previously stated, New (23) has thoroughly reviewed the methodology and theoretical basis of *in vitro* rat embryo culture. The particularly interested reader is referred to this source for further study.

Thorough analysis of the cultured embryos on a points system, developed by Brown and Fabro (4), results – in our laboratory – in a developmental score of 42·30 after culture as opposed to 44·56 *in vivo* (Table 2). The total protein and nucleic acid levels are reduced and this corresponds with some earlier observations made by New (22). He showed that the minutae of the culture technique employed could give rise to quite wide variations in protein levels after 32 h of culture whereas the levels up until that time remained identical to *in vivo* levels. Between-laboratory comparisons are, therefore, difficult to achieve. No abnormal embryos were present in either our *in vivo* or our *in vitro* series.

The period of culture during which the rat embryo grows comparably *in vivo* and *in vitro* lies between 9½ and 11½ days of gestation (23). This corresponds to the development and closure of the neural tube and the method is, therefore, of particular relevance to the study of neural tube defects. It may be argued that species difference is important in extrapolating animal results to man (see p. 2) but in this context Wilson's (34) comments are of importance,

> . . . it is an accepted principle of comparative embryology that species differences in form and structure become less striking as earlier embryonic stages are examined . . . it is an interesting but largely unstudied possibility that interspecies metabolic differences are also minimal in the embryo. In this eventuality differences in teratologic susceptibility would have to be attributed mainly to differences in placental transfer and in maternal metabolism rather than in the embryo's reaction to the agent.

In the absence of sufficient experimental work it would be premature to accept Wilson's speculation as fact but the remarkably constant, undifferentiated appearance of early embryonic cells under the electron micro-

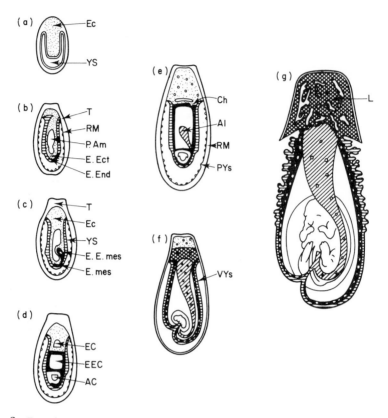

Fig. 3. Development of the extra-embryonic membranes of the rat. (a) At 6·5 days' post-fertilization. The ectoplacental cone has grown so that the inner cell mass has become invaginated into the yolk sac cavity. The latter is now horse-shoe shaped. (b) At 8 days; formation of the proamniotic cavity. A proamniotic cavity has appeared in the inner cell mass extending into the ectoplacental cone. The endoderm covering the sides of the ectoplacental cone is called the visceral layer of the yolk sac endoderm and in contrast to the parietal layer that is separated from the trophoblast only by an acellular layer known as Reichert's membrane, is highly pinocytic. The ectoplacental cone and the embryonic region at its apex are together known as the egg cylinder. (c) At 9 days gastrulation is well advanced. Mesoderm has migrated from the embryonic area into the region of the ectoplacental cone where ("pushing" the extra-embryonic ectoderm ahead of it) it begins to subdivide the proamniotic cavity. A small extra-embryonic coelom continuous with the embryonic coelom has developed. (d) At 9·5 days; division of the proamniotic cavity into three. The extra-embryonic mesoderm with its contained extra-embryonic coelom has grown right across the proamniotic cavity, and three cavities are apparent in the egg cylinder. They are an upper epamniotic cavity, a middle extra-embryonic coelom and a lower amniotic cavity. (e) At 10 days; development of the allantoic bud. The embryo has begun to form head and tail folds. The allantois, an outgrowth of the endoderm in the tail fold covered by allantoic mesoderm, is growing into the extra-embryonic coelom.

scope and the proven late development of liver and other enzymes in embryogenesis as well as the undoubtedly sound basis of the biological theory of recapitulation make the assumption a reasonable one to work with unless proven otherwise.

Shepard *et al.* (26) showed that the early rat embryo derives its energy from glucose, that there is a relative lack of oxygen dependence and low activity of the terminal electron transport system. The Krebs cycle does not appear to function to an important extent until 11½ days so throughout the culture period energy is derived principally from glycolysis and the pentose-phosphate shunt. Lactate accumulates in the culture medium (Al-Alousi, personal communication) and if the culture medium is repeatedly used glucose is eventually reduced to a level at which growth is not sustained. At this point the effectiveness of the serum can be re-established by replenishing glucose to normal levels but not by addition of lactate or pyruvate. From what has been said previously it is probable that this pattern of energy production is ubiquitous among mammals though the timing of the change-over from glycolysis to oxidative phosphorylation may vary with species.

At this stage it is pertinent to discuss embryonic nutrition during neural tube development in more specific detail (see Beck (1) for review). In everyday usage "the placenta" in Eutherian mammals is a chorio-allantoic structure in which interchange between embryo and mother takes place across a "placental membrane" interposed between the embryonic and maternal circulations. This form of nutrition is called haemotrophic; before

---

The epamniotic cavity has collapsed; its original lower wall consists of extra-embryonic ectoderm and non-vascularised mesoderm, thus forming the chorion. (f) At 11·25 days; early chorio-allantoic placenta. The allantois has fused with the chorion and a labyrinthine chorioallantoic haemochorial placenta is established. The embryo has turned so that it is now convex dorsally and has become invaginated into the extra-embryonic coelom (this is sometimes incorrectly referred to as the yolk sac cavity). (g) At 16 days to full term; disappearance of parietal yolk sac and Reichert's membrane. The parietal layer of the yolk sac, Reichert's membrane, the adjacent trophoblast and attenuated decidua capsularis are resorbed and the visceral layer of the yolk sac is exposed to the cavity of the uterus. Ec ectoplacental cone; Ys yolk sac cavity; T trophoblast; P.Am proamniotic cavity; E.Ect embryonic ectoderm; E.End embryonic endoderm; E. mes. embryonic mesoderm; EC epamniotic cavity; EEC extra-embryonic coelom; AC, amniotic cavity; Ch, chorion; Al allantois; R.M. Reichert's membrane; PYs parietal yolk sac wall; VYs, visceral yolk sac wall; L, chorioallantoic placental labyrinth. The visceral yolk sac endoderm is essentially the organ responsible for histiotrophic nutrition in the rat and in all other rodents so far examined. Its cells absorb biopolymers in solution which have passed through the parietal yolk sac wall (or are secreted directly into the uterine lumen after 16·5 days of pregnancy). Haemotrophic nutrition possibly *begins* to function at 11·5 days when the allantois has established the beginnings of a labyrinthine *haemochorial* placenta.

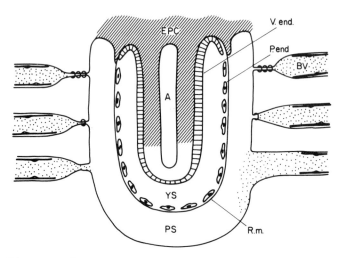

Fig. 4. Diagram to show relatively static blood in the blood sinus which is present in the trophoblast immediately surrounding the parietal yolk sac. Blood vessels entering and sometimes leaving the "lake" are relatively constricted (after Merker and Villegas (21a), with permission).

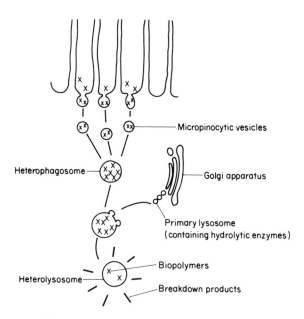

Fig. 5. Simplified diagrammatic representation of lysosomal breakdown of macromolecules. Recycling of secondary lysosomes is not shown; neither is the GERL concept of lysosomal formation.

Table 1. Results of morphometric analysis of the rat embryo endoderm.

Area of the egg cylinder	Day 9·5		Day 11·5	
	In vivo	*In vitro*	*In vivo*	*In vitro*
Visceral yolk sac endoderm				
Volume density	15·82 ± 0·51	16·61 ± 0·59	10·68 ± 0·21	11·20 ± 0·64
Surface density	0·58 ± 0·02	0·58 ± 0·02	0·49 ± 0·05	0·51 ± 0·02
Embryonic endoderm				
Volume density	2·26 ± 0·12	2·20 ± 0·18	–	–
Surface density	0·21 ± 0·01	0·18 ± 0·02	–	–

Each value is the mean ± s.e. (mean) for 6 embryos. Volume density represents the percentage of the total cytoplasmic volume occupied by the vacuolar system. Surface density represents the surface area of the vacuolar system as a proportion of the cytoplasmic volume. (from Gupta *et al.*, 1982).

it can be established considerable organogenesis must have occurred because the embryonic heart must be sufficiently developed to perfuse the fetal side of the placenta. Before this stage the embryo uses the endocytic properties of the extra-embryonic membranes to break down local uterine macromolecules; this is defined as histiotrophic nutrition. Some degree of histiotrophic nutrition persists in all species well after the onset of haemotrophic nutrition.

In the rat, the switchover from histiotrophic to a largely haemotrophic form occurs at 20–25 somites just after completion of the neural tube and closure of the posterior neuropore. This also coincides with the point at which the standard embryo culture technique ends, i.e. at 11½ days – see above. In man the beginning of haemotrophic nutrition occurs at 22–24 days (about 5 somites) at which stage the anterior neuropore is just closing while the posterior neuropore closes about two days later. A timetable of switchover from histiotrophic to haemotrophic nutrition in various species is given by Beck (2).

The fortuitously convenient nature of rat histiotroph makes it particularly suitable for the study of the nutritional requirements of the neurulating embryo. By crossed immuno-electrophoresis Huxham (personal communication) has found it possible to demonstrate that yolk sac fluid (i.e. the processed histiotroph produced after endocytosis and digestion of maternal plasma by the extraembryonic membrane known as the visceral yolk sac endoderm) contains about 12 major serum proteins. The overwhelming majority of plasma proteins endocytized by the yolk sac are, therefore, broken down to amino-acids by the lysosomal system of these cells (8).

Table 2. Culture of 9·5 day rat conceptuses for 48 hours in 100% rat serum (1). 100% human serum supplemented with glucose, final concentration 3 mg/ml (2). 90% human serum supplemented with glucose and 10% rat serum (3). Grown *in vivo* (4). From Lear et al. (in press).

Experiment	Mean yolk sac diameter (mm) ± s.e. (mean)	Mean crown-rump length (mm) ± s.e. (mean)	Mean somite no. ± s.e. (mean)	Mean morphological score ± s.e. (mean)[b]	Protein	Total nucleic acid
1	3·93 ± 0·072 (n = 49)	3·27 ± 0·047 (n = 49)	25·00 ± 0·45 (n = 49)	42·30 ± 0·20 (n = 49)	177 ug ± 10·39 (n = 23)	23·88 ± 0·90 (n = 28)
2	3·38[a] ± 0·15 (n = 45)	3·13[c] ± 0·05 (n = 45)	24·50 ± 0·23 (n = 45)	37·24[a] ± 0·57 (n = 45)	169 ug ± 8·52 (n = 30)	13·2 ± 0·48 (n = 18)
3	4·01 ± 0·062 (n = 40)	3·52[a] ± 0·054 (n = 40)	25·23 ± 0·17 (n = 40)	42·25 ± 0·26 (n = 40)	255 ug[a] ± 8·20 (n = 21)	50·27[a] ± 1·57 (n = 15)
4	—	3·72[a] ± 0·003 (n = 33)	26·94[c] ± 0·022 (n = 33)	44·56[c] ± 0·025 (n = 33)	362 ug[a] ± 11·28 (n = 16)	65·3[a] ± 1·99 (n = 17)

[a] Significant at $P < 0.001$ when compared with 1. [b] Determined using the method described by Brown and Fabro (1981). [c] Significant at $P < 0.05$ when compared with 1. n = number of conceptuses.

Further work in our laboratory has shown that inhibition of yolk sac endocytosis by trypan blue (32) or disturbance of intracellular digestion by a specific chemical known as leupeptin which acts by inhibition of cathepsins B H and L (3) both lead to embryonic malformation *in vitro* of which a large proportion are neural tube defects. Presumably this is because the embryo is deprived of essential nutrition. As well as the digestive properties of the rat extra-embryonic membranes we have also demonstrated by means of gold markers in conjunction with electron microscopy that a small number of specific macromolecules cross the yolk sac unchanged in special structures known as coated vesicles (13). Finally, by means of crossed immunoelectrophoresis as well as by radioactive precursor studies we have been able to demonstrate that cells almost certainly of yolk sac origin (which, unlike those of the embryo, are fully differentiated) secrete specific macromolecules (e.g. alphafetoprotein) into the yolk sac fluid presumably for use by the embryo (Huxham and Beck, in preparation). This confirms the work of Dziadeck who localized the production of alphafetoprotein to the yolk sac in the mouse conceptus.

In an important paper published in 1979, Cockroft (6) dialysed rat serum against glucose free buffered salt solution thereby removing the glucose, amino acids and vitamins from it. By systematic supplementation experiments he found that glucose was the only energy source that allowed growth to recommence (see above). He further showed that pantothenic acid, riboflavin, i-inositol and folic acid were also necessary for normal development. The implications of this experiment go far to confirm the results of Smithells' (29) supplementation studies quoted above.

Recently Al-Alousi and I (unpublished) have examined the effects of allowing rat embryos to stay in culture beyond 48 h. The results have been of some interest; the embryo dies and is absorbed but the yolk sac continues to expand and after 8 days of culture (with four media changes and daily gassing with 20% O_2, 5% CO_2 and 75% N_2) reaches a diameter of 2 cm containing 600 μl of yolk sac fluid (Fig. 6). This fluid is, in fact, processed histiotroph and is able to enhance the growth promoting properties of exhausted serum when the glucose level is appropriately adjusted. Al-Alousi (personal communication) has shown that the junctional complexes between the epithelial cells of the "giant yolk sac" remain intact and the vacuolar system looks normal under the electron microscope. Preliminary analysis of the contained fluid by two-dimensional thin layer chromatography suggests the presence of many, but *not* all, of the essential amino acids and by polyacrylamide gel electrophoresis, at least five major and three minor protein bands. The giant yolk sac is, therefore, a model for looking at *processed histiotroph* in large quantities and should prove an important model for the further investigation of embryonic nutrition.

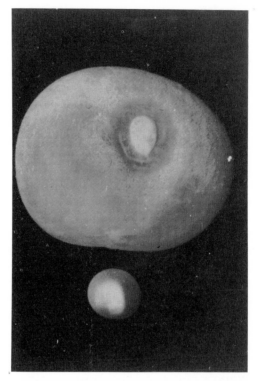

Fig. 6. Below: rat yolk sac with contained embryo at 11·5 days (after 48 hours of culture from 9·5 days) × 2·5. Above: rat yolk sac allowed to expand in culture for eight days beyond the usual time of harvesting at 11·5 days. Equivalent, therefore, to a 19·5 day yolk sac *in vivo*. The ectoplacental cone is facing the viewer × 2·5.

The Use of Embryo Culture in the Study of Teratogenesis

The immediate advantage of whole embryo culture applied to teratological problems is that the method provides an opportunity of separating the initiating causes into those active on the mother and those directly active on the conceptus. Thus, McGarrity *et al.* (21), working in our laboratory, have tested the teratogenic effects of sodium salicylate by comparing on the one hand the fate of embryos grown in serum to which sodium salicylate had been added to give serum levels commensurate with the optimum terato- genic dose and, on the other, the fate of embryos grown in serum from salicylate-treated rats. No effective difference was demonstrated and it was concluded that salicylates had a direct action on the conceptus. This obser- vation casts considerable doubt on suggestions by Goldman and Yacovac (9) that salicylate teratogenicity is mediated by maternal central nervous system catecholamine release. By contrast Fantel *et al.* (7) using the same technique have shown that teratogenic levels of cyclophosphamide *in vitro* are without effect on the embryo unless S-9 maternal liver fractions and co-factors for mono-oxygenation were added. This indicated that maternal biotransformation was a necessary prerequisite of cyclophosphamide teratogenicity. Similar conclusions were reached by Klein *et al.* (14), who also demonstrated the *in vitro* teratogenicity of cadmium.

Chatot *et al.* (5) grew rat embryos on pure human serum pretreated by the method of New and supplemented with glucose to the levels normally found in rat serum. This group has also published the preliminary results of a study in which the teratogenicity of some anti-convulsants and smoking was shown by *in vitro* rat embryo culture in human serum. If their work is shown to be repeatable its application is considerable. We have already suggested that metabolic similarities between the rat and human embryo are probably great at early developmental stages. This leaves only differences in the way that human trophoblast and the rat yolk sac process histiotroph as a significant factor in comparing the early human developmental system and the *in vitro* rat culture system performed on human serum. Experiments in which rat embryos are grown in the serum of smokers and non-smokers, in those exposed to lead or cadmium and in serum from women who are infertile or have repeated abortions without a known cause could thus yield results of fundamental interest. The important point to remember here is that testing rat embryos on human serum means that the *human maternal metabolism* is also tested in such a system. Differences occurring between experimental conditions (say, the effect on embryonic growth of the serum of smokers) and control conditions (the progressive changes, if any, which occur in explants on serum from individuals who are giving up smoking) are reflections of changes in the *maternal* metabolism following cessation of smoking.

Unfortunately, we have been unable to repeat the results of Chatot *et al.* (5). Tables 2 and 3 from work in our laboratory show the effect of growing rat embryos on 100% (glucose supplemented) human serum compared with 90% human serum supplemented with 10% rat serum and glucose. The effects are dramatic and growth of the embryo in the rat serum supplemented medium is as good, if not better than, in pure rat serum. The reasons for this are not easy to pin down but, as previously mentioned, it has been shown by Huxham and Beck (13) that certain macromolecules cross the yolk sac unchanged and it may be that traces of some of these are essential for normal rat development. Clearly this pin-points a potential weakness in growing rat embryos on *pure* human serum for such factors would be missing in such a medium. It should be mentioned finally that rat embryos will not grow in 10% rat serum and 90% buffered saline solution. It may, therefore,

Table 3. Comparison of abnormalities found after culture in 100% human serum and 90% human serum supplemented with rat serum.

9½ day rat embryos grown in:	Macroscopic appearance	
	100% human serum n = 36	90% human serum 10% rat serum n = 30
Anaemia (on gross inspection)	36	Nil
Major abnormalities[a]	15	Nil

[a] 8 had retarded neural tube closure. 4 had multiple major abnormalities. 3 were incompletely turned. From Reti *et al.* (25a).

be concluded that our method of culture on rat supplemented human serum may well retain the advantages of growth on pure human serum without exhibiting the uncertainties of unacceptable embryonic development in controls.

Though I have made a case for the value of *in vitro* experiments in the investigation of teratogenesis in general, and neural tube defects resulting from nutritional causes in particular, it is important not to leave the subject without introducing a cautionary note. The indiscriminate extrapolation of *in vitro* results to the *in vivo* situation is clearly unacceptable. Maternal toxicology will greatly modify an effect found *in vitro* and each situation must be assessed separately in this light. Maternal factors may be clearly defined by the method described above and then, if no special effect due to either yolk sac or trophoblastic factor is demonstrable, guarded – but often far-reaching – conclusions are possible.

Present Knowledge of Embryonic Nutritional Requirements *in Vitro*

The absolute requirement for adequate glucose and vitamin levels if embryonic growth is to take place *in vitro* has already been referred to. It is also not possible to grow normal embryos in media in which serum protein digestion is inhibited by leupeptin and supplementation with amino acids has been attempted. The reason for this is not clear but, as previously mentioned, it may be that certain amino acid transport mechanisms necessary for transfer of these substances across the yolk sac epithelium are inadequate. Alternatively, it may be that a sufficiency of amino acids to sustain growth cannot be maintained unless they are supplied to the yolk sac in "concentrated" protein form.

Al-Alousi (personal communication) has repeatedly grown rat embryos in the same batch of serum until the latter will not support growth even though its glucose and vitamin levels are replenished and toxic metabolites (lactate and pyruvate) are dialysed away. He concludes that besides vitamins, proteins, minerals and glucose the embryo also requires traces of specific growth factors. This possibility has already been mentioned and is made the more likely by Al-Alousi's (personal communication) success in reconstituting much of the growth potential of his exhausted serum by mixing it with yolk sac fluid derived from giant yolk sacs (see above).

Conclusions

Smithells (27) has cogently summarized the epidemiological situation concerning human neural tube defects and diet, particularly with respect to the role of vitamins. Apart from his conclusion that "hopefully these data may also move the balance of teratological research effort away from the creation of defective animals towards the creation of whole human beings" his arguments are persuasive. Perhaps enough has been said in this communication to refute emotive statements concerning the value of some aspects of teratological research for, if taken seriously, they may prejudice the future of important basic scientific work.

Passing from the epidemiological data, there is strong *in vivo* and *in vitro* evidence in Hurley's (12) review and Cockroft's (6) paper to support the importance of the role of vitamins in early mammalian development. The problem of the clinical work using Pregnavite forte F (Bencard) is that certain constituents of this polyvitamin preparation may be without effect. This is now difficult to show in human trials because of the obvious ethical difficulties of leaving out a vital supplement if each constituent is tested in turn. No such constraint governs *in vitro* animal experiments and it is in this field that findings such as those described by Smithells *et al.* (28) may be amplified and refined to a point at which it is possible to make an acceptable judgement concerning the probable situation in the human. Then specific clinical trials would be less unacceptable in ethical terms.

Acknowledgements

Much of the work (referred to as personal communication) reported here is, as yet, unpublished. The relevant experiments have been carried out by Doctors Gulamhusein, Reti, Gupta, Al-Alousi, Huxham and Misses Gaukroger, Clarke, Lear and Bulman.

I am grateful to Miss Reeve for careful preparation of the manuscript. This work was supported by grants from the M.R.C., from the National Fund for Research into Crippling Diseases and from an anonymous donor. I am grateful to all these for their support.

References

1. Beck, F. (1981). Comparative placental morphology and function. *In* "Developmental Toxicology" (C. A. Kimmel and J. Buelke-Sam, eds) pp. 35–54. Raven Press, New York.
2. Beck, F. (1982). Lessons from studies in animals for the evaluation of human risk from teratogenic agents. *In* "Advances in Pharmacology and Therapeutics II" (H. Yoshida, Y. Hagihara and S. Ebashi, eds) Vol. 5, pp. 17–28. Pergamon Press, Oxford.
3. Beck, F. and Lowy, A. (1982). The effect of cathepsin inhibitor on rat embryos grown *in vitro*. *J. Embryol. exp. Morphol.* **71**, 1–9.
4. Brown, N. A. and Fabro, S. (1981). Quantitation of rat embryonic development *in vitro*: a morphological scoring system. *Teratology* **24**, 65–78.
5. Chatot, C. L., Klein, N. W., Piatek, J. and Pierro, L. J. (1980). Successful culture of rat embryos in human serum: Use in detection of teratogens. *Science* **207**, 1471–1473.
6. Cockroft, D. L. (1979). Nutrient requirements of rat embryos undergoing organogenesis *in vitro*. *J. Reprod. Fertil.* **57**, 505–510.
7. Fantel, A. G., Greenaway, J. C., Juchau, M. R. and Shepard, T. H. (1979). Teratogenic bioactivation of cyclophosphamide *in vitro*. *Life Sci.* **25**, 67–72.
8. Freeman, S. J., Beck, F. and Lloyd, J. B. (1981). The role of the visceral yolk sac in mediating protein utilization by rat embryos cultured *in vitro*. *J. Embryol, exp. Morph.* **66**, 223–234.
9. Goldman, A. S. and Yacovac, W. C. (1965). Teratogenic action in rats of reserpine alone and in common with salicylate and immobilisation. *Proc. Soc. exp. Biol. Med.* **118**, 857–862.
10. Gregg, N. M. (1941). Congenital cataract following German measles in the mother. *Trans. Ophthalmol. Soc. Aust.* **3**, 35–46.
11. Gupta, M., Gulamhusein, A. P. and Beck, F. (1982). Morphometric analysis of the visceral yolk sac endoderm in the rat *in vivo* and *in vitro*. *J. Reprod. Fertil.* **65**, 239–245.
12. Hurley, L. S. (1977). Nutritional deficiencies and excesses. *In* "Handbook of Teratology" (J. G. Wilson and F. C. Fraser, eds) Vol. I, pp. 261–308. Plenum Press, New York and London.
13. Huxham, M. and Beck, F. (1981). Receptor mediated coated vesicle transport of rat IgG across the 11·5 day *in vitro* rat yolk sac endoderm. *Cell Biol. Int. Rep.* **5**, 1073–1081.
14. Klein, N. W., Vogler, M. A., Chatot, C. L. and Pierro, L. J. (1980). The use of cultured rat embryos to evaluate the teratogenic action of serum: cadmium and cyclophosphamide. *Teratology* **21**, 199–208.
15. Klein, N. W., Plumefisch, J. D., Carey, S. W., Chatot, C. L. and Clapper, M. L. (1982). Evaluation of serum teratogenic activity using rat embryo cultures. *In* "Culture Techniques" (D. Neubert and H.-J. Merker, eds) pp. 67–81. Walter de Gruyter, Berlin.
16. Laurence, K. M., James, N., Miller, M. and Campbell, H. (1980). Increased risk

of recurrence of pregnancies complicated by fetal neural tube defects in mother receiving poor diets and possible benefit of dietary counselling. *Br. med. J.* **281**, 1592–1594.

17. Laurence, K. M., James, N., Miller, M. H., Tennant, G. B. and Campbell, H. (1981). Double-blind randomised control trial of folate treatment before conception to prevent recurrence of neural tube defects. *Br. med. J.* **282**, 1509–1511.

18. Lenz, W. (1961). Kindliche Missbildungen nach Medikament während der Gravität. *Deutsch. Med. Wochenschr.* **86**, 2555–2556.

19. Lenz, W. and Knapp, K. (1962). Thalidomide embryopathy. *Arch. Environ. Health* **5**, 100–105.

20. McBride, W. G. (1961). Thalidomide and congenital malformations. *Lancet* **ii**, 1358.

21. McGarrity, C., Samani, N., Beck, F. and Gulamhusein, A. P. (1981). The effect of sodium salicylate on the rat embryo in culture: an *in vitro* model for the morphological assessment of teratogenicity. *J. Anat.* **133**, 257–269.

21(a). Merker, H. J. and Villegas, J. (1970). Electronenmikros Kopishe Untersuchungen zum Problem des Stoffaustausches zwischen Mutter und Keim bei Rattenembryonen des Tages 7–10. *Z. Anat. Entw Gesch.* **131**, 325–346.

22. New, D. A. T. (1976). Techniques for assessment of teratologic effects: Embryo culture. *Environmental Health Perspectives* **18**, 105–110.

23. New, D. A. T. (1978). Whole-embryo culture and the study of mammalian embryos during organogenesis. *Biol. Rev.* **53**, 81–122.

24. New, D. A. T., Coppola, P. T. and Cockroft, D. L. (1978). Improved development of rat head fold embryos in culture resulting from low oxygen and modification of culture serum. *J. Reprod. Fertil.* **48**, 219–222.

25. Palmer, A. K. (1981). Regulatory requirements for reproductive toxicology: theory and practice. *In* "Developmental Toxicology" (C. A. Kimmel and J. Buelke-Sam, eds) pp. 259–287. Raven Press, New York.

25(a). Reti, L., Bulman, S. and Beck, F. (1982). Culture of 9½ day rat embryos in human serum supplemented and unsupplemented with rat serum. *J. exp. Zool.* **223**, 197–199.

26. Shepard, T. H., Tanimura, T. and Robkin, M. (1970). Energy metabolism in early mammalian embryos. *Dev. Biol. Suppl.* **4**, 42–58.

27. Smithells, R. W. (1982). Neural tube defects: Prevention by vitamin supplements. *Pediatrics* **69**, 498–499.

28. Smithells, R. W., Sheppard, S., Schorah, C. J. *et al.* (1980). Possible prevention of neural tube defects by periconceptional vitamin supplementation. *Lancet* **i**, 339–340.

29. Smithells, R. W., Sheppard, S., Schorah, C. J., Seller, M. J., Nevin, N. C., Harris, R., Read, A. P. and Fielding, D. W. (1981). Apparent prevention of neural tube defects by periconceptional vitamin supplementation. *Arch. Dis. Child.* **56**, 911–918.

30. Warkany, J. and Nelson, R. C. (1940). Appearance of skeletal abnormalities in the offspring of rats on a deficient diet. *Science* **92**, 383–384.

31. Warkany, J. and Schraffenberger, E. (1944). Congenital malformations induced in rats by maternal nutritional deficiency. VI: Preventive factor. *J. Nutr.* **27**, 477–484.

32. Warkany, J., Roth, C. B. and Wilson, J. G. (1948). Multiple congenital malformations: a consideration of aetiologic factors. *Pediatrics* **1**, 462–471.

33. Williams, K. E., Roberts, G., Kidston, E. M., Beck, F. and Lloyd, J. B. (1976).

Inhibition of pinocytosis in the rat yolk sac by trypan blue. *Teratology* **14**, 343–354.

34. Wilson, J. G. (1973). "Environment and Birth Defects." Academic Press, London and New York.
35. Wilson, J. G. (1977). Current status of teratology. *In* "Handbook of Teratology" (James G. Wilson and F. C. Fraser, eds) Vol. I, pp. 47–74. Plenum Press, New York and London.

Commentary

Michael Laurence: This is an interesting account of a new approach to the study of the way environmental and especially nutritional changes can influence rat embryo development at the stage of neural tube closure and the changeover from histiotrophic to haemotrophic nutrition. It also suggests that because of the similarities of the rat to the human embryo, conclusions formed from such experiments can be highly relevant.

Unfortunately, Professor Beck only briefly touches on a number of experiments critical to the present problem, namely that glucose deprivation retards rat embryo development and that pantothenic acid, riboflavin, i-inositol and folic acid are essential for normal development at this stage. There is no whole embryo culture work quoted in which either energy deprivation or absence of vitamins actually seems to have produced faulty closure of the neural tube, or any work showing changes in the basic requirements of any of these substances which take place at the time of neural tube closure or the changeover from histio- to haemotrophic nutrition. There is no reference to any work being carried out on the way heavy metals or zinc, etc. influence the closure of the neural tube. In short, we are given information as to how rat embryo culture might be used to elucidate the problem under discussion only. Finally, embryo culture may well in future sort out the embryo's end of the maternal-fetal axis but it will probably not help greatly in sorting out the way the maternal genotype influences embryonic development.

Author's reply: New (3) deals with energy deprivation at length. He quotes various sources indicating that the early post-implantation embryo relies upon glycolysis and the pentose-phosphate shunt for its energy source and that after $10\frac{1}{2}$ days of development the contribution of the Krebs cycle begins to rise.

Our own unpublished work (Al-Alousi, in preparation) shows quite unequivocally that repeated culture of embryos in unchanged serum depletes glucose levels and raises lactate levels until growth becomes impossible. In cultures where glucose has already been substantially depleted but is still not quite exhausted poor growth is often accompanied by NTD and other defects. Laurence is substantially correct in saying that no whole embryo culture work has yet been done to show NTD resulting from vitamin defect, though abstracts have appeared from Klein's laboratory and our own work is well advanced.

Cockroft (1) has shown that embryos can be grown normally for a further 42 h if explanted at 12·5 or 13·5 days if the fetal membranes are opened up and oxygen is allowed direct access to the embryo. At 13·5 days haemotrophic nutrition *in vivo* is well under way. By modifying the experimental conditions Cockroft has presumably made enough oxygen available to the embryo to allow the Krebs cycle to function until the embryo is too large to receive all its requirements by the restricted vitelline circulation. Thus after 42 h it ceases to grow because the much more comprehensive haemochorial chorio-allantoic placental interface becomes indispensible.

Klein *et al.* (2) showed that rat embryos cultured in serum from rats treated with cadmium ($2·13 Cd^+/kg$) produced a majority of "exencephalic" embryos when serum 8 h after injection was used. To my knowledge zinc has not yet been tried in this system.

One of the particular strengths of the embryo culture system is the ability to investigate maternal genotypic influences on embryonic development. It is possible to culture the rat embryos from the primitive streak stage in the sera of disparate mothers of various genotype. A good controlled experiment can, therefore, be set up where the only variable is the genotype of the "mother" producing the culture serum. Indeed, the advantage of this system over the conventional whole animal experiment is the possibility of testing maternal and embryonic factors independently.

1. Cockroft, D. L. (1973). Development in culture of rat fetuses explanted at 12·5 and 13·5 days of gestation. *J. Embryol. exp. Morph.* **29**, 473–483.
2. Klein, N. W., Vogler, M. A., Chatot, C. L. and Pierro, L. J. (1980). The use of cultured rat embryos to evaluate the teratogenic activity of serum: Cadmium and Cyclophosphamide. *Teratology* **21**, 199–208.
3. New, D. A. T. (1978). Whole embryo culture and the study of mammalian embryos during organogenesis. *Biol. Rev.* **53**, 81–122.

John Edwards: Animal studies do not allow the assertion that the "insult to human populations will be low". They merely allow man to be protected from that group of insults which would also injure experimental animals.

Author's reply: I have stated that the *probability* of insult to human populations will be low. The meaning of my remark has, perhaps, been misinterpreted.

Dick Smithells: Beck makes the following two statements: ". . . it is unlikely . . . that attention to diet alone . . . will eliminate posterior rachischisis in man completely" and ". . . if nutritional defects are a factor in causing neural tube abnormalities . . . they may equally well help to produce other malformations".

I believe the first statement is certainly true and the second probably true. In this connection it is interesting to note:

(a) The change in social class distribution of NTD in the UK over a period of 25 years (Figs 7 and 8).
(b) The secular change in NTD incidence in recent years, *not* attributable to prenatal diagnosis (Fig. 9 and Table 4).
(c) The social class gradient in selected defects including NTD (Fig. 10).
(d) The secular change in incidence of selected defects including NTD (Table 5).

Chatot gave a paper to the Teratology Society meeting at French Lick, Indiana, in June 1982 extending this work. The results appear to have a direct bearing on the subject matter of this Workshop. The published abstract follows:

We have previously reported the use of rat embryo cultures to detect teratogenic activity in serum from epileptics receiving single anticonvulsant drug treatment. Teratogenic activity was detected in 18 of 21 (82%) Tegretol samples, 36 of 48 (75%) Dilantin samples, 15 of 21 (71%) valproic acid samples, 17 of 29 (58%) Phenobarbital samples and 4 of 8 (50%) untreated epileptic samples. We now report on the ability to overcome the teratogenic effects in some cases by supplementing the serum with vitamins and amino acids prior to use in culture. When serum samples, which were initially teratogenic, were supplemented, reduced teratogenicity was observed in 17 of 23 (74%) Dilantin

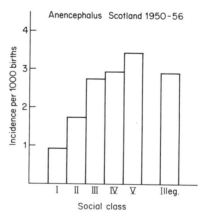

Fig. 7. Anencephalus, Scotland 1950–6.

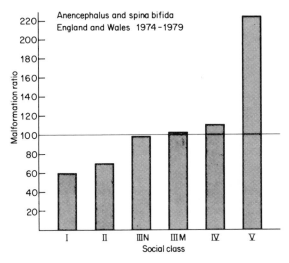

Fig. 8. Anencephalus and spina bifida, England and Wales 1974–9.

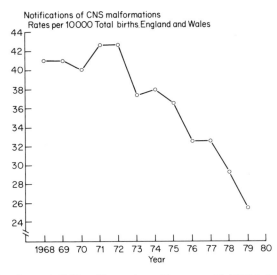

Fig. 9. Notifications of CNS malformations. Rates per 10 000 births, England and Wales.

Table 4.

Year	Notifications of CNS malformations	Legal abortions for suspected CNS malformations
1971	3378	53
1972	3129	51
1973	2553	45
1974	2452	34
1975	2227	73
1976	1915	81
1977	1870	124

England and Wales.

samples, 7 of 9 (78%) Phenobarbital samples, 6 of 12 (50%) Tegretol samples, 0 of 6 (0%) vaproic acid samples and 2 of 3 (67%) untreated epileptic samples. Supplementation produced increases in embryo protein content and improvement in embryo morphology including closure of open neural tubes, correction of eye defects and improvement of partial or dorsiflexed curvature. In 13 samples that responded to supplement, sufficient serum was available to show that different samples required specific and different portions of the vitamin and/or amino acid supplements to overcome the teratogenic activity.

I wonder why Beck cannot repeat the results of Chatot and Klein?

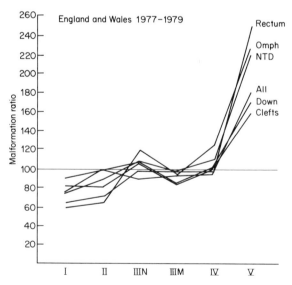

Fig. 10. England and Wales 1977–9.

Table 5. Notifications of malformations.

Malformation category	1973	1979
All babies	195·3	209·2
CNS	37·3	25·4
Cleft lip and/or palate	14·4	13·3
Cardiovascular	10·6	11·8
Limbs	67·4	85·0

Rates per 10 000 births, England and Wales.

Beck makes a spirited defence of animal teratological studies whilst cautioning (p. 10) that "the indiscriminate extrapolation of *in vitro* results to the *in vivo* situation is clearly unacceptable". His wish to refute emotive statements concerning the value of some aspects of teratological research is clearly directed at me (and others, perhaps) as in the preceding sentence he appears not to share my hope that "the balance of teratological research effort" might move "away from the creation of defective animals towards the creation of whole human beings".

I believe it is fair to say that there is no evidence so far that animal teratology studies have led to the prevention of any human malformations, nor is any animal species a reliable predictor of the human response. The difficulty here is that if animal tests suggest that a drug has teratogenic potential it will never reach the market and the hypothesis cannot be tested. I am also critical of the *enormous* doses used in many animal teratology studies (e.g. vitamin A given to rodents in a dose equivalent to 40 000 000 iu daily in man).

Having said that, I believe animal teratology has a vital part to play in elucidating mechanisms, and in the present context, though sad to spoil a good argument, I think rat embryo culture in human serum offers a superb opportunity to clarify the role of vitamins.

Peadar Kirke: Beck mentions that one of the problems in using Pregnavite forte F is that certain constituents of this multivitamin preparation may be without effect. He goes on to point out the difficulty of testing each constituent in human trials. The randomized control trial now underway in Ireland and the proposed United Kingdom Medical Research Council trial will clarify the position to a considerable extent. Two of the treatment groups in each trial are folate alone and the combination of the remaining constituents of Pregnavite forte F. Thus, these trials will answer the question of whether folate alone or the combination of the other constituents alone reduces the recurrence risk of neural tube defect. If these trials should show a dramatic effect for the multivitamin preparation (without folate) alone, then it would be very difficult to test each constituent in further human trials. In such a situation, *in vitro* and *in vivo* animal studies would be important in attempting to identify the efficacious constituent.

I fully agree with Professor Beck in his view that *in vivo* and *in vitro* animal experiments are an essential part of research into human congenital defects.

Author's reply: I strongly believe that *now* is the best time to do *in vitro* studies. The big human trials are in their infancy and will take some time to complete. The *in vitro* studies using human serum as laid out in my manuscript can be quickly performed especially since a great deal of serum from normal and NTD bearing mothers is acceptable.

Results of the *in vitro* studies would probably provide very strong evidence for the detailed planning of parts of the (inevitable) human study.

Mary Seller: I think the statement about the implications of Cockroft's experiment for Smithell's studies is incorrect. These experiments cannot *confirm* the human work. They are not comparable, for Smithells *et al.* took women "at risk", i.e. those with a genetic predisposition to producing children with an NTD, supplemented them with multivitamins and reduced the recurrence in the offspring. Cockroft took normal rat embryos without a genetic predisposition to NTD, cultured them through neurulation and withdrew individual vitamins, and also added some.

Further, other agents too, added or withdrawn at this stage in culture and, for example, imbalance of oxygen in the gaseous phase will also produce NTD. The vitamins are not specific in producing NTD.

Regarding the experiments of Chatot *et al.*, it is stated that if their work is repeatable, "its application is considerable", but we are not told what the results are, i.e. what it is that may be significant?

Author's reply: I have in fact written "*go far*" to confirm the human work; who is to say that Smithells' group were genetically predisposed and who is to say that the individual embryos in Cockroft's experiments were not genetically pre-disposed?

The significance of Chatot's experiments is that *rat* embryos will grow in *human* serum and, therefore, any response will be to *human* toxicity or metabolic changes. Surely such a departure is significant if a repeatable response to a human toxin is shown?

Don Naismith: One cannot deny the value of teratological research using such elegant techniques as those described by Dr Beck. If the human embryo, like the rat embryo, depends on glycolysis rather than oxidative phosphorylation for energy production until after the development and closure of the neural tube, then a role for riboflavin deficiency in the aetiology of NTD is difficult to envisage.

Author's reply: I have amended my manuscript to make it clear that *some* activity of the Krebs cycle is possible. Therefore, the role of riboflavin deficiency in the aetiology of NTD is not *completely* excluded though I quite agree with Dr Naismith that it is unlikely. I have done this in view of Cockroft's (1) findings quoted on p. 33 of my chapter. Nevertheless there are weaknesses in Cockroft's method. One wonders, for example, how success-ful his dialysis methods were in removing *all* the relevant vitamins from the serum he used as culture mediums.

1. Cockroft, D. L. (1979). Nutrient requirements of rat embryos undergoing organo-genesis *in vitro*. *J. Reprod. Fertil.* **57**, 505–510.

Norman Nevin: This paper is a comprehensive review of the use of whole embryo rat culture in teratology and highlights the possible application of this technique in elucidating the role of environmental factors in the aetiology of congenital malformation. Both the *in vivo* and *in vitro* approaches have the advantage in that manipulations of the environment and genetic compo-nents can be undertaken in a way in which it is impossible to do so in man. Undoubtedly, Beck's and Seller's animal models have an important part to play in elucidating the pathogenesis of neural tube defects.

Several points in the paper require attention:

(1) The introductory sentence of the paper is misleading. It is clear that even after "the 'rediscovery' of Mendel's work", many workers still considered birth defects to be determined largely by environmental factors (1, 2).

(2) "There is reason to believe, therefore, that if nutritional defects are a factor in causing neural tube abnormalities when active early in gestation, they may equally well help to produce other malformations at later periods" (p. 2). It may be relevant to this suggestion that several midline defects (in a non-syndromal association) have been observed more frequently among individuals with NTDs than in the population. Recently Czeizel (3) demonstrated a greater-than-chance association between neural tube defects, oral clefts, omphalocele, and diaphragmatic hernia. In addition, these "schisis" abnormalities

were noted in 3·7% of sibs of propositi. In his data there were 26 cases of anencephaly with cleft lip with or without cleft palate. Lemire *et al.* (4) also confirmed a high incidence of cleft palate among 68 fetuses with anencephaly.

(3) Little data is provided which would help elucidate the role of vitamins in the prevention of NTDs. I look forward to future work in which the rat embryo culture will be employed to study the effect of vitamins and trace-metals on the closure of neural tube defects. However, a difficulty with the rat embryo culture model is that no account is taken of the maternal genotype on the development of the embryo.

1. Birch-Jensen, A. (1949). Congenital deformities of the upper extremities. Commission: Andelsbogtrykkeriet i Odense and Det danske Forlag.
2. Warkany, J. (1971). "Congenital Malformations". Notes and Comments Year Book Medical Publishers, Chicago.
3. Czeizel, A. (1981). Schisis-association. *Am. J. Med. Genet.* **10**, 25–35, 1981.
4. Lemire, R. J., Beckwith, J. B. and Warkany, J. (1978). "Anencephaly". Raven Press, New York.

Author's reply: I have already referred to Cockroft's (1) work. This author showed the necessity of certain vitamins; the effect of cadmium is given in my reply to Professor Laurence's comments; the effect of the maternal genotype is also given in my reply to Professor Laurence's comments. It is perhaps the central strength of this method that New's technique has been modified to allow us to use *human* serum and thus to vary the maternal factors be they genotypic or phenotypic.

1. Cockroft, D. L. (1979). Nutrient requirements of rat embryos undergoing organogenesis *in vitro*. *J. Reprod. Fertil.* **57**, 505–510.

Ian Leck: In connection with the suggestion that if nutritional defects are a factor in causing neural tube defects in man, they may well help to produce other malformations also, it may be relevant that cleft lip as well as neural tube defects was among the defects described by Thiersch in the offspring of women given the folate antagonist aminopterin in early pregnancy (2), and that in a very recently reported trial of periconceptional multivitamin administration to women who had previously borne children with cleft lip, the recurrence rates were 1·2% in 84 births to women who accepted the vitamin supplement and 7·3% in 206 births to women who declined it (3). However, one would expect the scope for prevention by manipulating the environment to be less in cleft lip than in neural tube defects, since the latter show far more striking spatial and temporal variations within ethnic groups than the former (1).

1. Leck, I. (1981). Epidemiological aspects of paediatrics: insights into the causation of disorders of early life. *In* "Scientific Foundations of Paediatrics", 2nd edition. (J. A. Davis and J. Dobbing, eds) pp. 947–979. Heinemann, London.
2. Thiersch, J. B. (1952). Therapeutic abortions with a folic acid antagonist, 4-aminopteroyl-glutamic acid (4-amino P.G.A.) administered by the oral route. *Am. J. Obstet. Gynecol.* 1298–1304.
3. Tolarova, C. M. (1982). Periconceptional supplementation with vitamins and folic acid to prevent recurrence of cleft lip. *Lancet* ii, 217.

Nicholas Wald: It would be helpful if Professor Beck could indicate whether the *in vitro* investigations he describes can clarify whether or not folic acid or other vitamin deficiencies can cause neural tube defects. The paper suggests that they can, but I do not think that the relevant data and arguments are presented.

Author's reply: Dr Wald is quite correct in stating that neural tube defect has as far as I know not yet been described in detail in vitamin deficient whole embryo cultures. What has been shown by Cockroft (1) and our own group is failure of growth and abnormal structure which latter has not yet been analysed. Recently Chatot (2) read a paper (June 1982) at the American Teratology Society meeting in which Klein's group claim to have ameliorated the teratogenic action of anticonvulsants by vitamin and amino acid supplementation. Neural tube closure is specifically mentioned.

1. Cockroft, D. L. (1979). Nutrient requirements of rat embryos undergoing organogenesis *in vitro*. *J. Reprod. Fertil.* **57**, 501–510.
2. Chatot, C. L. *et al.* (1982). American Teratology Society Meeting, French Lick, U.S.A.

Editor's note: See also Appendix III.

Chris Schorah: The *in vitro* system described by Beck is more adaptable than whole animal studies (2) because it offers the possibility of continuous monitoring of the effects that constituents in the medium, which are easily varied, have on the developing fetus. However, as I understand the technique described, it does not assess the influence of maternal factors on the induction of fetal malformations. There appear to be no maternal components present in the system. Maternal/fetal interrelationships may be of crucial importance to the development of the neural tube (2). Indeed, Beck outlines the importance of the critical period in the changeover of nutrient supply of the fetus from histiotrophic to haemotrophic nutrition and it is of particular interest that this occurs in the human at about the time of closure of the neural tube (1). Environmental factors could affect the timing of this changeover as could both maternal and fetal genetic traits. In some animals genetic problems leading to delay in the transfer from histiotrophic to haemotrophic nutrition could be overcome or modified by adequate nutrition. In others, with a different genetic influence, the same nutritional supplement may be totally ineffective. It is this critical changeover in the type of nutrient from histiotrophic to haemotrophic supply that may be difficult to study in the animal model described by Beck.

And advantage of the *in vitro* model described, is that species differences are said to be minimized in early embryonic growth. Vitamin C has been implicated in the aetiology of NTD (3) in man, but adult rat and man do not obtain this compound from the same source. I know of no evidence to suggest that the situation is different in the embryo, although it has been suggested that, unlike the adult, guinea pig embryos can synthesize vitamin C (4).

I would not wish to suggest that the animal model outlined is of little importance in the study of NTD. Arguments could be made for the application of such models to a detailed examination of the way the neural tube closes or fails to close and what factors are important at the various stages. This is important information, but I remain sceptical that such studies will yield detailed information about the environmental factors which influence the prevalence of NTD in man.

1. Beck, F. (1982). The use of whole embryo culture of the rat in the experimental study of human birth defects. *ibid.*
2. Seller, M. J. (1982). Maternal nutritional factors and neural tube defects in experimental animals. *ibid.*
3. Smithells, R. W., Sheppard, S. and Schorah, C. J. (1976). Vitamin deficiencies and neural tube defects. *Arch. Dis. Childh.* **51**, 944.
4. Yew, M. S. (1975). Biological variation in ascorbic acid needs. *Ann. N.Y. Acad. Sci.* **258**, 451.

Author's reply: As mentioned in connection with Professor Laurence's comments the technique has been developed precisely to investigate maternal differences on embryonic development. As then mentioned, it is possible to culture rat embryos from disparate mothers (rat *or* human). A controlled experiment can, therefore, be set up where the *only* variable is the genotype of the "mother" producing the culture serum – be she rat or human. Indeed, the advantage of this system over the conventional whole animal experiment is the possibility of testing maternal and embryonic factors independently.

The dimensions of the rat conceptus are such that culture is easy until 11½ days of development. The rat neural tube closes at $11^1/_3$ days. Using special techniques (hyperbaric oxygen, opening of the yolk sac) growth can be extended to $13^1/_2$ days so that in appropriately controlled experiments any NTD must certainly be due to the culture serum. It is true that the human neuropores are finally closed only at 28 days while human placental tertiary villi begin to have circulating blood in them at 23 days. It is only on this last point that the rat model fails to mirror the human system exactly. Though this matter must be borne in mind it applies only to the final regions of neural tube closure. I feel that the majority of effects will have been detected previously.

I have been unable to find any precise information concerning the synthesis of vitamin C by early somite rat and human embryos and I doubt whether any timed study exists.

Felix Beck's general comments: I feel it most important to stress that *in vitro* studies will be maximally effective if they are carried out *now*. As I point out in my reply to Dr Kirke's comments I believe that they could in a relatively short period of time provide important information which could conceivably modify the methods used in carrying out the human trial. The result might be a considerable speeding up of the whole process because the human studies could ask the right questions early on. Additionally a more efficient human study would of course have important revenue consequences.

Prevention of Neural Tube Defects by Vitamin Supplements

R. W. SMITHELLS

*Department of Paediatrics and Child Health,
University of Leeds, Leeds*

Introduction

The importance of good maternal nutrition to normal fetal development has been accepted as self-evident for a long time, but scientific investigation of this field has appeared on the scene relatively recently. In the clinical arena, credit must be paid to Mellanby (8) for his continuing emphasis on the relevance of maternal nutrition to pregnancy outcome. On the experimental front, the classic paper of Hale (3) (on pigs without eyeballs) and the long-term work of the Cincinnati team headed by Warkany (16) demonstrated that under some circumstances nutritional deficiencies in pregnancy (notably of vitamins) could cause congenital malformations.

Because of a proper reluctance to translate animal experiments to human problems, a recognition that many of these studies involved dietary manipulations of a degree quite unattainable in man under ordinary circumstances, and a belief that in developed countries nobody was significantly malnourished, the early animal work was not thought relevant to the study

This paper also appears in "Nutrition in Pregnancy", published by the Royal College of Obstetricians and Gynaecologists, March 1983.

of human malformations. However, before the twentieth century was half-way through there were a few straws in the wind. Epidemiological studies of human malformations, especially of neural tube defects (NTD), showed a striking social class gradient which required an explanation (2). Nutrition was one of several obvious candidates for consideration. Aminopterin, a folic acid antagonist, was found to be teratogenic in humans (15). A study of folate status (using the Figlu test*) at the *end* of pregnancy showed a striking difference between mothers of NTD infants and controls (4).

Epidemiological studies of NTD have revealed interesting secular trends in incidence. Over the last decade or two incidence has fallen in many developed countries.

The relatively low incidence of NTD in some developing countries has been interpreted by some as evidence against a nutritional contribution to NTD causation. However, the populations concerned have a different genetic constitution, and diets deficient of protein and energy are not necessarily deficient of vitamins (see comments by Naismith, p. 68).

Diet in Pregnancy

Although nutrition involves a far wider range of physiological functions than mere eating, diet is clearly an important component. Studies of diet in pregnancy are relatively numerous: studies of diet in *early* pregnancy are relatively rare. Methodology presents many problems. The techniques most often used are (1) 24-h recall, and (2) weighed and recorded intakes. The first has the advantages of simplicity and – provided the subjects are not forewarned of the interview – the fact that the survey does not influence that which is being surveyed. The disadvantages are that recall may be inaccurate and/or incomplete; the method can only be used for the immediately preceding 24 h, and this may have been in some respect an atypical day; and that quantities can only be assessed in very crude terms. The advantages of the weighed and recorded intake, which should last 7 days (or, if shorter, include a week-end) lie in the completeness and accuracy, permitting calculation of mean daily intakes of individual nutrients. The disadvantages are that it may influence eating patterns, is relatively expensive, and a lot of supervision is needed by subjects of poor intelligence and education.

In relation to the current nutrition/NTD debate, two surveys have been published in the UK. Smithells *et al* (10) studied 195 women in the first trimester of pregnancy by weighed dietary records normally covering 7 days. Intakes appreciably lower than those recommended were associated with lower social class, maternal age under 20 years, smoking, and pregnancy

* Urinary excretion of FormIminoGLUtamic acid after oral loading dose of histidine.

sickness. When the mean intakes of social classes I + II were compared with those of classes III + IV + V, the differences were highly significant for all nutrients. At the time of the study there were no published UK values for the folate content of foods. This information has subsequently become available, and low folate intakes show the same associations as do low intakes of other nutrients. Comparison of folate intakes is difficult because (a) analytical techniques in the past have almost certainly underestimated folate content, and (b) there is no general agreement on folate requirements and at present there is no published UK recommendation about this.

The only nutrient for which intakes were almost universally well below current recommendations was vitamin D.

Laurence *et al.* (6) used a questionnaire to assess first-trimester dietary intakes retrospectively in 174 mothers of NTD infants. Mothers were asked to provide details of their diets when they were not pregnant and during the first-trimester of all their pregnancies, including those ending in the birth of NTD infants. The NTD births occurred between 1954 and 1969. Assuming that the questionnaires were issued in 1969/70 (the paper does not make this clear), mothers appear to have been asked to recall their dietary habits at least 6–9 months previously, and at most 15 years or more previously. Diets were assessed as good, fair or poor. Of 174 pregnancies associated with NTD, first-trimester diets were assessed as good in 17 (9·8%) and poor in 92 (52·9%). In the other 123 pregnancies, diets were assessed as good in 23 (18·7%) and poor in 37 (30·1%). These differences are highly significant.

In this study dietary counselling was given to 103 women before their next pregnancy but not to a further 71 women, the groups being determined on a geographical basis. Dietary intake was assessed by interview during the first 6 weeks of the next pregnancy and was found to be much better in the counselled mothers (36·7% good diets) than in the uncounselled (16·9% good diets). The incidences of NTD in these pregnancies were 3% in the counselled group and 7% in the uncounselled, but all these recurrences occurred in women whose diets had been prospectively rated to be poor.*

Although the technique for assessing diet in previous pregnancies in the Laurence study is open to substantial criticism, these two dietary studies allow three conclusions:

(1) There is a marked social class difference in first-trimester intakes of all nutrients.
(2) Dietary habits can sometimes be influenced by counselling.
(3) In South Wales, NTD recurrence is associated with poor first-trimester maternal diet.

---

* The South Wales study of folate supplementation (7) was carried out concurrently with the dietary study, so some of the counselled mothers *and* some of the uncounselled received folic acid 2 mg b.d.

Vitamin Chemistry in Pregnancy

First trimester blood levels of selected vitamins were measured in the first trimester of pregnancy in over 900 women by Smithells *et al.* (11), and associations sought (1) with social class and (2) with NTD birth. Two hundred and forty-five social class I and II mothers showed significantly higher mean levels than mothers of lower social class with respect to red cell folate, white cell vitamin C, red cell riboflavin and serum vitamin A, and a non-significantly higher mean level of serum folate.

Seven mothers (including the one described in the addendum to Ref. 10) gave birth to babies with malformations of the central nervous system – four with anencephaly, one with myelomeningocoele and hydrocephalus, one with meningocoele (normally classified as a neural tube defect but not involving neural tissue) and one with microcephaly (involving neural tissue but not normally classified as NTD). This group of mothers had significantly lower mean first-trimester levels of red-cell folate and white cell vitamin C. There was also evidence of riboflavin deficiency but not to the point of statistical significance. Subsequently vitamin B_{12} levels were estimated and found to be particularly low in the mothers of anencephalics (9).

Intervention Studies

The circumstantial evidence summarised above justifies intervention studies designed to reduce or eliminate the incidence or recurrence of NTD by dietary counselling and/or vitamin supplementation. The dietary counselling study of Laurence (8) suggested limited success. Vitamin supplementation studies have been undertaken on over 450 high-risk mothers by Smithells *et al.* (12, 13, 14), on 60 high-risk mothers by Laurence *et al.* (7) and on 43 high-risk mothers by Holmes-Siedle *et al.* (5).

Smithells et al. (13)

The subjects were women who had had one or more NTD infants, who were considering a possible further pregnancy but who were not pregnant at the time of recruitment. They were recruited predominantly through genetic counselling clinics, but also by referral from hospital consultants and general practitioners. All women meeting the above criteria were invited to join the supplementation study.

The supplement offered was Pregnavite forte F®, 1 tablet 3 times a day, which was chosen because it included folic acid, vitamin C, riboflavin (shown to be deficient in the biochemical study) and vitamin D (shown to be deficient on the dietary study). Furthermore, the dietary survey had shown a lower intake of *all* nutrients in lower social class mothers. Pregnavite forte F also contains vitamins B_1, B_6, nicotinamide, iron and calcium (but not zinc) (see Chapter 1, Table 1).

The regime advised was to start supplementation not less than 28 days prior to conception and to continue until the date of the second missed menstrual period.

The study was therefore *not* a placebo study (although this was the original intention), *not* randomized and *not* blind. Provisional results for Cohorts 1 and 2, by social class, are shown in Table 1.

Table 1. Vitamin supplementation study. Cohorts 1 and 2 (provisional).

Social class	Fully supplemented	Partially supplemented	Not supplemented
I	53	13	28
II	90	15	74 (4)
IIIN	58 (1)	13	48 (4)
IIIM	175 (2)	43	230 (10)
IV	47	16	78 (3)
V	13	2	15
Subtotal	436 (3)	102	473 (21)
Unclassifiable and Unknown	18	13	46 (3)
Total	454 (3)	115	519 (24)

Figures in brackets = NTD recurrences.

Laurence et al. (7)

The subjects were as in the Smithells *et al.* study.

The supplement offered was, on a random basis, either folic acid 2 mg b.d. or placebo b.d. The regime was to start when contraceptive precautions were stopped. Total duration is not stated.

Sixty women were allocated to the folate group and 51 to placebo. Serum folate was estimated at 6–9 weeks gestation. None of the placebo group had a level above 12 μg/l. Mothers in the folate group were divided into "compliers" or "non-compliers" according to whether their serum folate levels were above or below 10 μg/l. On this basis, 16 of 60 women were classified as non-compliers.

This study was therefore randomized (folate or placebo) and double-blind. Six pregnancies ended in NTD births, four in the placebo group and

two in "non-compliers" in the folate group, a combined recurrence rate of
$6/67 = 9\%$. There were no recurrences amongst 44 mothers judged to have
taken folate.

Holmes-Siedle et al. (5) (preliminary results)

Forty-three women were treated according to the protocol of Smithells *et al.*
There were no recurrences.

Problems Not Yet Fully Resolved

Does Vitamin Supplementation Prevent NTD?

Imperfections of study design compel a very careful scrutiny of results to
determine, if possible, whether the *apparent* protective effect of vitamin
supplementation is real, or whether selection bias and/or compliance problems could account for the results. Smithells *et al.* (13) considered four
possible interpretations:

(a) Women with "naturally" low recurrence risks selected themselves for
supplementation. The obvious factor worth considering is social
class, but place of residence and previous obstetric history could be
relevant. Careful scrutiny of these factors does *not* support the suggestion that confounding variables are responsible for the different
recurrence rates as between supplemented and unsupplemented
mothers.

The study was carried out at a time of secular decline in NTD
incidence which might be associated with a similar decline in *recurrence*
rate. In theory, the recurrence risk after one affected child could have
halved over 10 years. This leads to the possibility shown in Table 2.

Table 2.

Year	No. of mothers	Population recurrence risk	No. of recurrences	Recurrence rate in group
1970	400	5%	20	5%
1980	Supplemented 200 ⎱	2·5%	⎰ 0	0%
	Unsupplemented 200 ⎰		⎱ 10	5%

It is possible that something of this sort may have *contributed to* the low recurrence rate in supplemented mothers, but data from Northern Ireland, and the Cardiff study, suggest that any such contribution is small. The Yorkshire Regional Study, which aims to recruit for supplementation *all* eligible women in a large population who have had a NTD birth since 1 January 1977, will also help.

(b) Supplemented women aborted more NTD fetuses spontaneously than did unsupplemented women. There is no evidence to support this.

(c) The effect is real, but is attributable to some factor other than vitamins. There is no evidence to support this.

(d) Vitamins have a protective effect. This is not only the most straightforward interpretation: it is entirely consistent with all the circumstantial evidence outlined above.

Do Vitamin Supplements do any Harm?

The quantities of vitamins in Pregnavite forte F are identical with, or slightly less than, current US recommended daily intakes. There is therefore no possibility of vitamin overdosage unless the mother is taking large quantities from some other source. Laurence's folic acid dosage (4 mg daily) is about 10 times the WHO recommendation for pregnant women. There is no evidence that this is harmful although some women may not be able to tolerate it. (Did this contribute to the high non-compliance rate in the Cardiff study?)

Follow-up examination of babies in the Smithells study has so far showed no evidence of harm.

What Vitamins are Necessary and in What Dose?

We do not know. Dietary studies suggest that women on poor diets are short of *all* nutrients. Biochemical studies showed associations between NTD and low blood levels of folic acid, ascorbic acid and riboflavin. Other B vitamins were not measured. A multivitamin supplement is therefore nutritionally appropriate and in keeping with the experimental evidence. Laurence's study, using folic acid alone, raises the possibility that this may suffice. Comparative studies which will answer this question are in progress.

What Period of Pre- and Post-Conceptional Supplementation is Necessary?

This is not known, but see next section for evidence that pre-conceptional supplementation for at least 28 days makes sense.

What is the Mechanism of Action?

If the recognized indications for vitamin therapy are considered, they fall under three heads:

(a) Correction of dietary deficiency (e.g. nutritional rickets)
(b) Overcoming a metabolic block (e.g. vitamin D resistant rickets)
(c) Other (e.g. pyridoxin for pregnancy sickness)

In conditions featuring a metabolic block, vitamin doses well in excess of normal physiological needs are usually required to overcome it. However, folates deserve special consideration because of the forms in which they exist in the diet. It is conventional to distinguish between "free folate" (mono- di- and tri-glutamate) and polyglutamate. The latter must be broken down by intestinal folate conjugases before they can be absorbed. Conjugase deficiency (absolute or relative) would interfere with polyglutamate absorption, and this could be circumvented by a very modest dose of "folic acid" because the monoglutamate is used in vitamin pills.

We have devised a polyglutamate absorption test using a standardized chicken liver pâté. Preliminary studies have shown:

(1) Subjects with low baseline values for serum folate achieve small rises after ingestion of pâté: those with high baseline values achieve higher rises.
(2) After a period of supplementation, not only does the baseline increase, but the response to pâté does also. Baseline values and responses are higher after 28 days supplement (Pregnavite forte F) than after 7 days.
(3) Serum folate begins to fall as soon as supplements are stopped.
(4) RBC folate begins to rise about 2 weeks after beginning supplements, and continues to rise for about 2 weeks after discontinuance.

These observations, which confirm earlier studies by others, suggest that if an individual's folate stores are poor, they will be topped up before serum folate rises. Their flat polyglutamate absorption curves reflect *not* poor absorption but rapid transit from serum to stores. There is evidence that the placenta is an important store, and transfer of folate to the embryo may therefore only become generous after body stores *and* placenta are replete (1).

Apart from a few reported examples of folate conjugase deficiency of genetic origin there is so far no evidence of a metabolic problem in mothers of NTD infants, but more work is needed. If a dietary *deficiency* is postulated, multivitamin supplementation is logical.

What are the Practical Implications?

The reply to this question can only be "enormous and daunting". So far studies have been confined to preventing *recurrences*, which account for about 5% of NTDs. These mothers are likely to be more motivated than others, yet Laurence found 27% non-compliance. If vitamins work by correcting a dietary deficiency, the theoretical answer lies in improving diets by health education. Certainly this should be attempted, especially in schools, but will it work?

Preconception (prepregnancy) clinics offer the best hope and give an opportunity not only to discuss diet and/or to prescribe vitamins, but to discuss smoking and alcohol, to check rubella immunity status and to take other steps to safeguard fetal health.

This leaves the unplanned pregnancy unprotected. As many of these are "pill failures", possibilities include the incorporation of vitamins into oral contraceptives, or – perhaps better – vitamin pills to be taken on the days when oral contraceptives are omitted in each cycle.

Problems of Study Design

Epidemiologists and statisticians are understandably irritated by the deficiencies of many clinical studies. We would all like to meet their strict criteria but it is not always possible. The need for double-blindness, randomization and placebos needs to be considered in the context of vitamins and NTD.

Double-blindness

The patient is the embryo who does not know what pills his mother is taking. The closure of his neural tube cannot be influenced by the doctor's knowledge of the pills. The mother could conceivably exert some indirect effect as a result of knowing what she was having, but would that not be a placebo effect?

Randomization

Patients can only be randomized between two or more treatments *after* admission to a trial. It is highly desirable to avoid selection biasses. Laurence *et al.* were able to randomize; Smithells *et al.* were not. In the future, randomization between different vitamin supplements should be possible.

Placebo

A placebo group does not tell you *whether* something works or not. If it does work, it may tell you something about *how* it works. If the effect is shown to be *entirely* a placebo effect, a less expensive substitute for the treatment may be used. A demonstrated placebo effect is not a reason to withhold a demonstrated benefit.

Acknowledgements

I wish to acknowledge the help and collaboration of my co-workers: Dr Sheila Sheppard, Dr Chris Schorah and Mrs Jenny Wilde (Leeds); Dr Mary Seller (London); Professor Norman Nevin (Belfast); Professor Rodney Harris and Dr Andrew Read (Manchester); Dr Stanley Walker (Liverpool) and Dr David Fielding (Chester).

References

1. Baker, H., Frank, O., Deangelis, B., Feingold, S. and Kaminetsky, H. A. (1981). Role of placenta in maternal-fetal vitamin transfer in humans. *Am. J. Obstet. Gynecol.* **141**, 792–796.
2. Edwards, J. H. (1958). Congenital malformations of the central nervous system in Scotland. *Br. J. prev. Soc. Med.* **12**, 115–130.
3. Hale, F. (1933). Pigs born without eyeballs. *J. Hered.* **24**, 105–106.
4. Hibbard, E. D. and Smithells, R. W. (1965). Folic acid metabolism and human embryopathy. *Lancet* i, 1254.
5. Holmes-Siedle, M., Lindenbaum, R. H., Galliard, A. and Bobrow, M. (1982). Vitamin supplementation and neural tube defects. *Lancet* i, 276.
6. Laurence, K. M., James, N., Miller, M. and Campbell, H. (1980). Increased risk of recurrence of pregnancies complicated by fetal neural tube defects in mothers receiving poor diets, and possible benefit of dietary counselling. *Br. med. J.* **281**, 1592–1594.
7. Laurence, K. M., James, N., Miller, M. H., Tennant, G. B. and Campbell, H. (1981). Double-blind randomised controlled trial of folate treatment before conception to prevent recurrence of neural-tube defects. *Br. med. J.* **282**, 1509–1511.
8. Mellanby, E. (1933). Nutrition and child-bearing. *Lancet* ii, 1131–1137.
9. Schorah, C. J., Smithells, R. W. and Scott, J. (1980). Vitamin B_{12} and anencephaly. *Lancet* i, 880.
10. Smithells, R. W., Ankers, C., Carver, M. E., Lennon, D., Schorah, C. J. and Sheppard, S. (1977). Maternal nutrition in early pregnancy. *Br. J. Nutr.* **38**, 497–506.
11. Smithells, R. W., Sheppard, S. and Schorah, C. J. (1976). Vitamin deficiencies and neural tube defects. *Arch. Dis. Child.* **51**, 944–950.

12. Smithells, R. W., Sheppard, S., Schorah, C. J., Seller, M. J., Nevin, N. C., Harris, R., Read, A. P. and Fielding, D. W. (1980). Possible prevention of neural tube defects by periconceptional vitamin supplementation. *Lancet* **i**, 339–340.
13. Smithells, R. W., Sheppard, S., Schorah, C. J., Seller, M. J., Nevin, N. C., Harris, R., Read, A. P. and Fielding, D. W. (1981). Apparent prevention of neural tube defects by periconceptional vitamin supplementation. *Arch. Dis. Child.* **56**, 911–918.
14. Smithells, R. W., Sheppard, S., Schorah, C. J., Seller, M. J., Nevin, N. C., Harris, R., Read, A. P., Fielding, D. W. and Walker, S. (1981). Vitamin supplementation and neural tube defects. *Lancet* **ii**, 1425.
15. Thiersch, J. B. (1952). Therapeutic abortions with a folic acid antagonist, 4-aminopteroyl glutamic acid (4-amino P.G.A.) administered by the oral route. *Am. J. Obst. and Gynaec.* **63**, 1298–1304.
16. Warkany, J. and Nelson, R. C. (1941). Skeletal abnormalities in the offspring of rats reared on deficient diets. *Anat. Record.* **79**, 83–100.

Commentary

Chris Schorer:

The multivitamin intervention studies; self selection and bias. The results of the intervention trials summarized by the reports of Smithells and Nevin, are persuasive and suggest a real reduction in recurrence of neural tube defect brought about by vitamin supplementation. The major criticism is that because the trials were not double-blind, randomized and placebo-controlled, a group of women of low recurrence unwittingly selected themselves for supplementation.

The only factors which are known to affect recurrence of NTD are the number of previous NTDs born to the mother, her social class and the area where she lives (4). Both unsupplemented and supplemented women in the study were chosen from the same areas and all were selected because NTD had affected at least one previous pregnancy. The social class distributions of the resulting groups were different, but differences in recurrence found between supplemented and unsupplemented women in social class IIIM, IV and V are still significant (7). Regional differences and bias introduced by the disproportionately large number of "controls" from Northern Ireland are also unlikely to have affected the outcome of the study, as shown by the significance of the results in Northern Ireland alone (Chapter 5). However, there remains the possibility that factors which affect the risk of recurrence and which have not yet been identified could have been under-represented in the supplemented group because of the process of selection. There are however arguments against this:

(1) The potato avoidance trial (5) did not unwittingly select patients at lower risk from a high risk group in spite of the commitment required of women in that study who had to avoid potato and potato products during their pregnancy. Such a protocol would have been more likely than the vitamin intervention trial to select the motivated woman and therefore the better cared-for pregnancy and produce a lower risk group. It did not. Equally important is the work of Laurence *et al.* (Chapter 4), who found recurrence at the expected rate (6·9%, Table 8) in a group of women who had received placebo supplements, but who were selected in a similar way to those receiving Pregnavite forte F supplements in the multicentre trial (7). If selection was responsible for the decreased recurrence in the multivitamin trial, Laurence, applying a similar selection procedure, should have found a recurrence rate of 0·7% in his placebo group.

It follows, therefore, that it appears difficult to select a group at substantially lower risk for NTD from a population at high risk by erecting selection hurdles that have to be negotiated by those of the invited population who succeed in complying with the protocol.

(2) If selection of a lower risk group for supplementation had occurred in the study, then provided that the control and supplemented groups together formed a substantial proportion of the total NTD recurrences in a given area, the controls should have had a higher rate of recurrence than would be expected. Of the regions involved in the multivitamin supplementation trial, the supplemented and control mothers in Northern Ireland are a very large proportion of the total NTD recurrences of the area. However, the recurrence rate in the Northern Ireland control group is 5·2% (Chapter 5, Table 9).

This is slightly less than the expected, for if the population *occurrence* rate averaged 0·44% during the trial (Chapter 5, Table 2, 1978–80) then *recurrence* should be 6·6% by calculation (square root of occurrence, ref. 1), or 6·2% by extrapolation (Chapter 6, Fig. 2). The Northern Ireland control group, therefore, shows no increase in recurrence risk and hence no evidence of a low risk supplemented group having been self selected from it.

One danger of concentrating on the bias, which does exist in the Pregnavite forte F trial, and assuming that this has led to self selection of a group of naturally low recurrence (Wald, general comments to the meeting), is that a real difference between the control and the supplemented is missed. This is that all supplemented women in the trial were planning a pregnancy. Unplanned pregnancy is not a known risk factor, but contraceptive practices between the supplemented and control groups would have been different and the supplemented women would be on average more prepared for pregnancy. They would, in short, have received periconceptional care in addition to vitamins. Jongbloet (2) has postulated that unplanned conceptions lead to increased prevalence of NTD because of damage to gametes. An assessment of the number of NTD recurrences in unsupplemented women who had planned their pregnancy as opposed to those who had not, would help resolve this criticism.

Important information which could support the damaged gamete theory is the very high recurrence (55%; 6 NTD out of 11 women) in women (Appendix to Chapter 4, Table 10 of Chapter 5) in the trials of multivitamin and folic acid (Chapters 3 and 5) who did not take vitamins before the 28th day of pregnancy. They were not women who were unable to take tablets reliably; they were simply unknowingly pregnant at the time of issue of the tablets or became pregnant before they asked for tablets. This could imply either an unplanned pregnancy or very variable menstrual cycles. There may be an important clue here to the aetiology of NTD, and prospective trialists may wish to adjust or monitor their trials to account for these observations.

Few would doubt the principle of using a randomized placebo-controlled trial to confirm the findings of the multivitamin intervention studies, but there will almost certainly be difficulties in the organization and the interpretation of the results of such studies. Future placebo-controlled trials will presumably use women at recurrence risk for NTD, but such groups are becoming aware of the protective nature of multivitamin supplements. Multivitamin preparations are freely available and recently preparations containing folic acid can also be acquired without prescription (6). It will therefore be necessary to make measurements of blood folic acid concentrations in both placebo and supplemented individuals in future placebo-controlled trials.

An additional problem faced by trialists, is the falling prevalence of NTD (Chapter 6). This not only makes it necessary to recruit more women into the trial, but if decreased prevalence is due to changes in environmental factors, it increases the possibility that genetic predisposition becomes more dominant in those who continue to have NTD. Seller (Chapter 1) describes the strong genetic influence, both maternal and fetal, on the incidence of NTD in the curly-tail mouse and the difficulty of modifying the prevalence of NTD in this species with nutrients other than vitamin A. It seems therefore probable that as the genetic factor becomes more predominant in the population at risk for NTD, it will be more difficult to reduce NTD by environmental influence. An alternative to the double-blind randomized placebo-controlled study would be to saturate an area of high "prevalence" with periconceptional vitamin supplements. By treating almost the whole population the problems of biased selection and ethical use of a placebo are avoided. The design and ethical problems of future studies underline the need for full analysis of the intervention trials already undertaken in order that all possible explanations for the findings of these studies can be investigated.

1. Edwards, J. H. (1982). Vitamin supplementation and neural tube deficits. *Lancet* **i**, 275.
2. Jongbloet, P. H. (1981). Declining incidence of neural tube defects. *Lancet* **ii**, 1291.
3. Kiely, M., Scott, B. and Bradwell, A. R. (1981). Zinc status and pregnancy outcome. *Lancet* **i**, 893.
4. Nevin, N. C., Johnston, W. P. and Merrett, J. D. (1981). Influence of social class on the risk of recurrence of anencephalus and spina bifida. *Develop. Med. Clin. Neurol.* **23**, 1.
5. Nevin, N. C. and Merrett, J. D. (1975). Potato avoidance during pregnancy in women with a previous infant with either anencephaly and/or spina bifida. *Br. J. Prev. Soc. Med.* **29**, 111.
6. Shaklee, (1981). "Product in formation; B-complex". Shaklee International, Milton Keynes.
7. Smithells, R. W., Sheppard, S., Schorah, C. J., Seller, M. J., Nevin, N. C., Harris, R., Read, A. P. and Fielding, D. W. (1981). Apparent prevention of neural tube defects by periconceptional vitamin supplementation. *Arch. Dis. Child.* **56**, 911.
8. Tamura, T., Shane, B., Baer, M. T., King, J. C., Margen, S. and Stokstad, E. L. R. (1978). Absorption of mono- and poly- glutamyl folates in zinc-depleted man. *Am. J. Clin. Nutr.* **31**, 1984.

Nicholas Wald: Most of my comments are given under General Comments (see Appendix I).

It is said that international studies have shown relatively low incidence in some developing countries, which some have interpreted as evidence against a nutritional contribution to NTD causation. It would be useful if this evidence could be presented in more detail, together with Professor Smithells' assessment of it. If he feels the evidence does not argue against a nutritional contribution what are the reasons?

Does Vitamin Supplementation Prevent NTD? It is stated that an explanation for the results of the human intervention study may be that women with a naturally "low recurrence risk" selected themselves for supplementation. Various factors were considered but "careful scrutiny of these factors does *not* support the suggestion that confounding variables are responsible for the different recurrence rates between supplemented and unsupplemented mothers". Unless this statement can be supported it should be deleted. If the recurrence risk of neural tube defects has been declining (as is suggested) the sort of problem Professor Smithells outlines would have occurred, but it is not clear which data from Northern Ireland and the Cardiff study suggest that it would only be small. What is the Yorkshire Regional Study? How will it help? It is stated that vitamins having a protective effect is not only the most straightforward interpretation of the results but is entirely consistent with all the circumstantial evidence. This view may be correct, but it does not answer the relevant question, which is: "Is there a plausible alternative explanation?" since if there is, we cannot tell if the vitamins are effective.

Can the Vitamin Supplements do Harm? The question is crucial but it is dismissed too readily. It has been argued that it is unimportant whether the vitamin supplementation is proven to be effective since the pills are bound to be safe and there is no reason not to automatically offer supplementation and give women the benefit of the doubt. Regrettably, however, there are many examples of medical treatments that were at one time thought to be completely safe but later were shown to produce harmful effects, some of them very serious. For example, the use of vitamin D to prevent rickets led to the production of hypercalcaemia and its serious consequences. Another example is the use of oxygen in the treatment of premature babies. This is a particularly relevant example since at one time oxygen was regarded as being so safe that it was impossible to give too much – a view which was only reversed after the realization that a number of infants became blind due to retrolental fibroplasia. The third example is the administration of diethyl-stilboestrol during pregnancy to prevent recurrent miscarriage. Again it was argued that female sex hormones were "normal" and one was simply supplementing a group who may have been deficient. Later it emerged that the treatment caused vaginal cancer in the daughters of the treated women.

Problems of Study Design Smithells says that "non-medical epidemiologists and statisticians are understandably irritated by the deficiencies of some clinical studies". The suggestion is that the criticisms are unnecessarily fussy and therefore unwarranted. This opinion, however genuinely felt, does not help resolve the problem and should be dropped unless supported scientifically.

The points raised in connection with "double-blindness" and the use of a placebo are obscure. There are, in trials, several reasons for using a placebo and for introducing "blindness"; in a randomized trial of vitamin supplementation in the prevention of neural-tube defects the reason would be to avoid selective self-medication. Insofar as this is accomplished, Smithells' statement that "A placebo group does not tell you *whether* something works or not. If it does work, it may tell you something about *how* it works" is incorrect. In fact the reverse is true.

The section headed "What are the Practical Implications?" (p. 61) begs the question regarding the therapeutic effect of the vitamins and possible toxicity. At present there is so much scientific uncertainty that the practical implications should be those concerned with the design and execution of future studies which will resolve the matter. This is not considered in this paper, or to any great extent in any of the others.

Author's reply:
The relatively low incidence of NTD in some developing countries. (a) The people have a different genetic make-up and therefore cannot be directly compared, and (b) although often short of protein and energy they are not necessarily short of folic acid or vitamin C (see comments by Naismith).

"Unless this statement can be supported it should be deleted". It is fully discussed in my reference (13).

Yorkshire Regional Study. I apologise for not explaining. The problem of selection bias could be largely overcome if 100% of women in a defined area, giving birth to NTD infants over a defined period, were recruited for vitamin supplementation. Although 100% is unattainable we are attempting to get as close as possible by making a positive approach to all eligible mothers resident in the Yorkshire Region and having had NTD babies since 1 January 1977. Controls will have to be historical, or contemporary in neighbouring regions.

The most straightforward interpretation. Is there a *more* plausible alternative explanation?

Vitamin toxicity. All vitamins except folic acid (in significant quantities) can be purchased without prescription in the UK. Folic acid is off prescription in many countries. If there is serious concern about their possible toxicity in "nutritional" doses the evidence should be put before the Committee on Safety of Medicines. Does Dr Wald think that chicken liver, fresh fruit and other rich sources of vitamins should be put on prescription?

"Blindness". "There are, in trials, several reasons for using a placebo and for introducing blindness". It would be helpful if Dr Wald would list them. If results with placebo = results with vitamins, the two treatments are either equally *effective* or equally *ineffective*. If results with vitamins are better than with placebo, the placebo may be doing good, but the vitamins are better (and vice versa).

Don Naismith: The case for a dietary deficiency in the aetiology of neural tube malformations has been convincingly put by Professor Smithells, with evidence from animal studies, the effects of an antimetabolite in man, food intakes of mothers considered at risk of having affected fetuses, and finally his own impressive intervention studies. He is to be congratulated on his use of the 7-day weighed food intake in the assessment of diet, a difficult and time-consuming exercise which provides the only credible information on what people actually eat.

Evidence of a gradient in nutrient intakes relating to social class confirms the findings of the National Food Survey Committee, published annually. However, his concern over the failure of a high proportion of mothers of low social class to achieve the recommended intakes of certain nutrients emphasizes the widespread confusion over the meaning and application of these values. The record of blood levels of vitamins in at-risk mothers was a logical confirmation of the dietary data and an essential starting point for identifying the nutrients most likely to be involved in the causation of NTD.

His finding that mothers from the lower social classes and those with fetuses with NTD had abnormally low tissue stores of both folic acid and vitamin C, as indicated by erythrocyte and leucocyte concentrations, is particularly interesting. In the average UK diet, approximately one third of the vitamin C is obtained from oranges which are also a relatively good source of folic acid compared with other common fruits. The diets of these mothers are characterized by a lack of green vegetables and citrus fruits, usually considered dispensable when food choice is limited by economic means. The richest dietary sources are endive (330 μg/100 g), spinach (140 μg/100 g) and brocolli (110 μg/100 g) which could be termed "middle class foods" and liver (140 μg/100 g) an educated choice.

The use of Pregnavite forte F was both ethical and pragmatic. An alternative approach would have been to choose a vitamin on the basis of its known biochemical functions. Of all the vitamins shown to be lacking in the diets of mothers with NTD fetuses, one only, folic acid, is known to be directly involved in cell multiplication (and hence morphogenesis); its most important function is in the synthesis of thymidylic acid for incorporation into DNA. The relationship noted between maternal plasma B_{12} and anencephaly may be explained by the role of this vitamin in the liberation of metabolically active tetrahydrofolate. Vegans, who have notoriously low plasma B_{12} concentrations are not known to be at risk in this respect. They do, in general, have high intakes of folic acid, as do most poorly nourished mothers in the developing countries whose diets are largely vegetarian.

When considering the mechanism of action of the vitamin supplement, Smithells rejected the notion of a "metabolic block" in the absence of any evidence, and "other mechanisms" were not discussed. We were left, therefore, with the "correction of a vitamin (folate?) deficiency". But how is deficiency defined and what is its nature? All mothers with very low intakes of folic acid have megaloblostic anaemia, the classical symptom of deficiency, but few have fetuses with NTD. There appears to be no doubt that the affected embryo is either deprived of an adequate supply of folate, or requires an abnormally high concentration of folate to enable the neural tube to close. It seems highly improbable that the developing placenta should fill its own stores (as suggested in this paper) before transferring folate to the embryo when the main purpose of this organ is to nourish the embryo. A metabolic block might, however, exist in the extra-embryonic membranes. Vitamins are transported from the maternal to the fetal circulation by elaborate and complex mechanisms designed to favour a unidirectional flow. Folate, for example, circulates in the maternal plasma mainly as methyltetrahydrofolate; in the mature placenta it is found mainly as a polyglutamate and in the fetal circulation as the formyl derivative (1). Assuming the developing placenta has the same metabolic activity as the mature placenta, then a defective enzyme could interrupt these interconversions at any one of the stages of transport. Alternatively, if the embryo synthesizes its own thymidylic acid rather than receiving the preformed nucleotide from the maternal circulation (or the placenta), then the block might reside in the embryo itself. Examination of the placentas of delivered fetuses with NTD might be rewarding.

1. Landon, M. J. (1975). *Clin. Obstet. Gynaecol.* **2**, 413.

Felix Beck: A very persuasive review amounting to the strongest possible circumstantial evidence that certain vitamin deficiencies (those of the "B" group being particularly suspect) are in some way connected with the genesis of neural tube defects in an "at risk" population.

Two pieces of evidence suggest that vitamin deficiency may be responsible for a considerable number of the neural tube defects occurring in the *general* population at large. These are:

(a) the fact that the condition is commoner in the Registrar-General's Social Groups III, IV and V rather than in I and II:

(b) that the incidence is falling possibly because of the better nutritional status of present-day pregnant women.

Neither of these rather general observations is in any way conclusive. Indeed, other observations suggest that environmental agents apart from vitamin deficiency, together with a greater or lesser genetic predisposition, can give rise to neural tube defects. For instance, the wide-spread production of NTD in various animal experiments resulting from treatment at appropriate times with teratogenetic agents as diverse as aspirin, ionizing radiations and trypan blue is well documented while in man geographically and racially-based differences in the incidence of neural tube defect also point to the likelihood that factors other than vitamin deficiency play a part in the pathogenesis of neural tube defect.

The implications raised by Smithells' work are clearly impressive. In assessing its full significance one would wish to know to what extent vitamin deficiencies produce other congenital defects when active at other times during gestation. No analysis of associated defects in the populations considered are given and if, indeed, they are absent then one would suspect a degree of specificity in the relationship between vitamin deficiency and neural tube formation which, if true, is in itself an interesting observation. Is (for example) the fetal alcohol syndrome related to vitamin deficiency (2, 3)?

There is much to be said both for, and against, the inception of such a study with a polypharmaceutical preparation such as Pregnavite forte F. Casting a wide net is clearly more likely to produce results but, by the same token, their interpretation becomes that much more difficult.

A seminal reference (1) is missing from the bibliography.

We cannot ignore the "placenta" during neural tube closure. The extra-embryonic membranes at this stage have important metabolic and transport functions.

1. Cockroft, D. L. (1979). Nutrient requirements of rat embryos undergoing organo-genesis *in vitro*. *J. Reprod. Fertil.* **57**, 505–510.

Norman Nevin: *Causes of NTDs.* Recently, it has been suggested (a recent paper in *J. Pediatrics* and a paper presented at the *Clinical Genetics Society* April 1982) that NTD may be part of the spectrum of abnormalities in the fetal alcohol syndrome. However, whether the NTD is due directly to the teratogenic effect of alcohol, or is due to an associated dietary deficiency, or is a result of a combination of both these factors remains uncertain.

Author's reply: *Vitamin deficiencies and other congenital defects.* In theory they might work for facial clefts (and see Tolarova (1)). First trimester vitamin levels in 7 mothers of babies with congenital heart lesions were normal (Chapter 3, ref. 13).

Specificity of vitamins for NTD. The secular decline in NTD in UK and elsewhere has not occurred with other malformations. (With respect, my bibliography was certainly *not* comprehensive.)

1. Tolarova, M. (1982). *Lancet* **ii**, 217.

Ian Leck: As usual, Smithells provides a clear, realistic and well-balanced appraisal of his subject. I sense that his commitment to the view that vitamin supplementation can prevent neural tube defects is increasing, but not beyond what I believe the evidence justifies. Apart from his use of the term "incidence" when "prevalence at birth" is what is meant (see my comment on Nevin's paper), the only aspect of his paper that troubles me is the section "Problems of study design". "The cry . . . for double-blind, randomized, controlled, placebo trials" is not confined to non-medical scientists as the first words of this section might suggest, but comes from distinguished medical people as well, as Cochrane's "Effectiveness and Efficiency" (1) demonstrates; and although I agree with Smithells that these criteria cannot always be met, his more specific comments about them do not seem to have been fully thought through, still less integrated into clear recommendations as to how future studies should be designed (but perhaps this is because he sees this as a task for the workshop itself). On the double-blind issue (p. 61), his wording suggests to me that because any effect on the offspring produced by a mother's knowledge of how she was being treated in a clinical trial would be a placebo effect, it would not matter, which seems a *non-sequitur*. He seems to dismiss matching of cases and controls (of which pairing is the simplest form, not an alternative to it) because without randomization it is less adequate than randomization alone (p. 61); but matching may sometimes be better than making no attempt to improve the comparability of treated and untreated cases when (as in Smithells' own intervention study), randomization is impossible, and even in a randomized study one may be able to improve comparability by putting similar individuals into pairs (or larger sets) and randomly allocating a different treatment to each member of the set. Lastly, including a placebo group in a trial is said not to show "whether something works" (p. 62), which seems like an oversimplification: it may be true if active treatment and placebo have the same outcomes, but surely not if outcome is significantly better with active treatment than without?

1. Cochrane, A. L. (1971). "Effectiveness and Efficiency: Random Reflections on Health Services" (the Rock Carling Fellowship, 1971). Nuffield Provincial Hospitals Trust, London.

Author's reply:
Incidence v. prevalence. We need to agree terminology although this may not be easy. We need terms for: (1) The proportion of embryos that fail to close their neural tubes. (2) As (1), minus spontaneous abortions (estimated by Bell to be 90%). (3) Proportion of viable infants (28 weeks gestation or

more) with NTD, which equals (2) minus therapeutic abortions. This, rather than (2), is the traditional "birth prevalence".

Trial design. I admit to having half a tongue in one cheek, but the precise purposes of randomization (which I accept as important), double-blindness and placebo deserve debate. Blindness of investigator and subject is advised in case knowledge of therapy influences outcome. *Does the Workshop believe that this is likely to influence neural tube closure?* The placebo helps to determine what part of an effect (if any is observed) is attributable to the action of treating, as distinct from the specific nature of the treatment. Matching in case-control studies *may* be better than non-matching provided the limits of matching are recognized and over-matching is avoided.

John Edwards: I do not think the only adequate trials are those involving randomization. Block trials, in which a group, defined by space and time, are exposed, and the change in incidence noticed, could be regarded as controlled but not randomized. Randomized trials may eliminate bias, but only at high cost in efficiency. (See also my comments on Chapter 4).

Norman Nevin: As I have been one of the research group involved with Smithells, I have few comments on his paper, which reviews the current status in the field of periconceptional vitamin supplementation in the prevention of NTDs.

He argues that as the study was carried out during a period of decline in the prevalence of NTDs that there could be also an associated decline in the recurrence rate. The family data from Northern Ireland would suggest that this is an unlikely explanation for the significant difference between the treated and untreated groups. In relation to this point Smithells states "The Yorkshire Regional Study will also help". Nowhere in his paper is there an explanation of this study. Could we have more information.

Do vitamins do any harm? This is an important point to which the Workshop should address itself. Follow-up of the babies in the Smithells *et al.* studies has been ongoing. Perhaps it would be worthwhile updating and expanding this section. I agree that to date, there is no evidence of harm or indeed any increased prevalence of other congenital abnormalities in the treated groups.

What vitamins are necessary? It is important to appreciate that as stated (p. 59) there is evidence of an association between NTDs not only for low levels of folic acid but also for ascorbic acid and riboflavin. The fact that Laurence (Chapter 4) has demonstrated an association with poor maternal diet would indicate a generalized nutritional deficiency rather than a single deficiency. Undoubtedly, the proposed Medical Research Council and Dublin studies will contribute an answer.

What period of pre- and post-conceptional supplementation is necessary? Is there sufficient data from those women who have been "partially" rather than "fully" supplemented to answer this question. From Seller's work on curly-tailed mice and vitamin A, timing is vitally important.

Could Smithells expand on the role of the placenta as an important folate store? This is important. Many early references on the nature of anencephaly have mentioned poor placentation.

Author's reply:

Folate and the Placenta. It is agreed that the placenta is not relevant to NTD. Nevertheless, the paper (Chapter 3, ref. 1) is interesting because it suggests that, contrary to the old "fetus-as-parasite" teaching, the embryo may be at the end of a long queue for B_{12}, folate and B_6.

Mary Seller: At the time of neurulation in the embryo, the placenta has not been established, so this fact about the placenta is irrelevant in the context of production of NTD, although it is relevant with regard to fetal nutrition in general and observations on maternal folate levels in pregnancy.

Peadar Kirk:

Does Vitamin Supplementation Prevent Neural Tube Defects? Smithells asks whether the effect of vitamin supplementation observed in his studies (19, 20) is apparent or real. The essential problem in interpreting these findings is the lack of comparability of the supplemented and unsupplemented groups. The detailed description of these groups illustrates how different they are (20). There are, for example, marked differences between the groups in social class and in previous obstetric history. We do not know whether the favourable outcome in the supplemented mothers is greater than might be expected for such a self-selected group. The only satisfactory method of obtaining comparable groups of mothers is by the process of random allocation.

An unbiased analysis of the results of Smithells *et al.* (19, 20) is not possible because of the failure to randomize.

There is a number of problems relating to data analysis in the published reports of the work of Smithells and his colleagues and I will comment on two of them here.

There is incomplete follow-up information on 34 of the 342 mothers recruited for supplementation; three moved from the area; 18 withdrew before conception; 13 withdrew mainly because of alleged side-effects of the tablets and it was not known if any was pregnant at the time of withdrawal (20). Of these 34 mothers one would like to know (a) how many subsequently became pregnant, and particularly, if this occurred within 3 months of stopping supplementation, and (b) whether there were any births with neural tube defects (NTD).

In the description of the study methods in the preliminary report it is stated that the control or unsupplemented group comprised women who were "either pregnant when referred to the study centres or declined to take part in the study" (18). In the expanded report those who declined to participate are not mentioned as being part of the unsupplemented group (20). It is important to establish whether the unsupplemented group included such mothers. To include them with the unsupplemented mothers is another form of the compliance bias referred to in my comments on Laurence's paper.

In summary, the findings of Smithells and his colleagues *suggest* that vitamin supplementation *may* reduce the risk of recurrence of NTD. The essential point to remember is that, because of the study's methodological shortcomings (5, 6, 12, 15, 21), the efficacy of the multivitamin preparation, Pregnavite forte F, has not been established.

I would like at this point to present some preliminary findings from a study conducted in Dublin (11) which make an important point. The aims of this study were to determine prevalence rates at birth and recurrence rates of NTD in the four main Dublin maternity hospitals (Table 3). During the period 1970–5, 129 238 babies were born in these hospitals and 840 of these had a NTD, giving a prevalence rate at birth of 6·5 per 1000 total births. The mothers of these affected infants were followed up to determine their subsequent reproductive history (up to the end of 1981) with particular

Table 3. Recurrence of NTD among women who had at least one affected infant born in the Dublin maternity hospitals in 1970–5.

Hospital	Prevalence of NTD at birth[a] 1970–1975	Outcome of subsequent pregnancy[b]			
		Number of women	Normal infants	Affected infants	Recurrence rate %
Coombe	6·5	185	167	19	10·22
National	6·0	157	158	1	0·63
Rotunda	6·3	130	128	6	4·48
St. James's	8·9	65	63	4	5·97
Total	6·5	537	516	30	5·49

[a] Per 1000 total births. [b] ≥28 weeks' gestation.

reference to the recurrence of NTD in the family. There was considerable variation in the recurrence rates between these four hospitals (Table 1). The striking difference between the National Maternity (0·6%) and the Coombe (10·2%) hospitals cannot be explained by diffences between the study mothers or between the total hospital populations in social and demographic characteristics or in previous obstetric history; case ascertainment was similar in both hospitals (11). A possible explanation is that these two groups of women differed in respect of factors unknown to us which influenced their risk of recurrence of NTD. The study illustrates the pitfalls of using research designs other than the randomized clinical trial (for example, treating mothers in one hospital and using those in another hospital as controls) to evaluate the efficacy of vitamin supplementation in high-risk women.

Do vitamin supplements do any harm? Pre- and periconceptional intervention is exciting and daunting. What is daunting is the realization that in offering mothers treatment around the time of conception and during early pregnancy, we are experimenting during the period of most rapid fetal organogenesis. How safe is this? Professor Smithells tells us that follow-up of the babies in his study showed no evidence of harm. In the final report of the first cohort of supplemented mothers the authors report the significant defects recorded at birth for the 182 babies of the fully supplemented mothers and the results of follow-up examinations at ages 5 months to 3½ years for 85 of these babies (20). More recently, Smithells has gone further on the question of safety of vitamin supplementation in stating "it is certain that, in proper doses, they (the constituents of Pregnavite forte F) do no harm" (17). One simply cannot feel secure about the safety of periconceptional multivitamin supplementation until at least several thousand babies have been examined at birth and, preferably, followed-up into childhood.

Does the literature point to any dangers of taking iron or vitamin preparations during pregnancy? To my knowledge there are no reports which present strong evidence implicating iron or vitamins in the aetiology of congenital abnormalities but there are papers which suggest the possibility of an association and I would like to mention some of these.

It is worth recalling the finding by Nelson and Forfar in their case-control study that vitamin and iron preparations were consumed during the first 8 weeks of pregnancy by a significantly higher proportion of mothers of babies with congenital abnormalities (13). Mothers of babies with major abnormalities were more likely than controls to have taken these preparations during the first 14 days of pregnancy but the differences between the cases and controls, based on very small numbers, were not statistically significant. In another case-control study of aetiological factors in NTD carried out in Winnipeg it was found that both vitamin and iron pills were consumed more by certain NTD groups (14). It is not clear from the report of this study whether the vitamin/iron consumption relates to the first trimester or the total pregnancy.

Smithells states that as the quantities of vitamins in Pregnavite forte F are identical with, or slightly less than, current US recommended daily intakes, there is little possibility of vitamin overdosage unless the mother is taking large quantities from some other source. I agree with this assessment but, should periconceptional vitamin supplementation become widely practised, there will be the problem of some mothers taking excessive doses of pre-scribed or non-prescribed vitamin preparations for a variety of reasons. One such mother was noted in the study of Laurence *et al.* (10). This mother admitted to the study team that she had not taken the prescribed folate tablets during early pregnancy but had taken a large number of them at 7 weeks' gestation (i.e. at the time of neural tube closure), just before the field worker was due to visit her. Her pregnancy ended at three months in a spontaneous abortion of an anencephalic fetus. Interestingly, there is also a case on record of an anencephalic fetus, terminated at 17 weeks, associated with maternal megavitamin therapy for psychiatric reasons during early pregnancy (2, 3). This patient was taking tablets of thiamine (100 mg), pyridoxine (100 mg), niacin (200 mg), ascorbate (200 mg) and brewer's yeast, all in variable quantity but at a minimum of four tablets of each per day for 6 months prior to conception and during the first 10 weeks of pregnancy. Seller mentions the report by Bernhardt and Dorsey of congenital renal anomalies occurring in a baby whose mother took very large doses of vitamin A throughout pregnancy (4).

There have been some conflicting reports on the possible teratogenicity of vitamin D. High doses of vitamin D have been correlated with aortic stenosis in rabbits (8) and humans (7). However, Antia *et al.* studied 15 children with this anomaly and found no association with maternal vitamin D excess (1). Also, Goodenday and Gordan reported on 27 normal children born to women who were hypoparathyroid and had to take an average of 107 000 IU of vitamin D daily throughout pregnancy to maintain normal serum calcium (9).

Periconceptional vitamin supplementation is unlikely to be harmful to mothers provided excessive intake is avoided and special cases (e.g. patients with renal disease) are appropriately supervised. However, in the event of a sizeable proportion of childbearing women taking vitamin supplements containing folic acid for prolonged periods, there is the possibility of mask-ing subacute combined degeneration of the spinal cord in cases of pernicious anaemia.

What vitamins are necessary and in what dose? The trials underway will answer the question of whether folate *alone* or a multivitamin preparation without folate (Pregnavite forte F in the Irish trial and a similar preparation in the proposed UK Medical Research Council trial) *alone* significantly reduces the recurrence of NTD. It is theoretically possible that an efficacious effect could be due to a synergistic interaction between folate and the constituents of the multivitamin preparation. In that situation only the combined preparation (Pregnavite forte F in the Irish trial) would be effective and mothers on folate or multivitamins (without folate) only would experience the expected recurrence rate of approximately 5%; both trials will detect such an effect provided that it is quite marked.

If the trials show that the multivitamin preparation alone is effective and should such a protective effect be large, it would be difficult from the ethical viewpoint to test the efficacy of the constituents in further trials on humans. As Smithells says, we do not know what dose of vitamins is necessary, assuming, of course, that the effect observed by Smithells and Laurence is confirmed in the trials underway. The trials may shed light on this if folate alone should prove to be the efficacious agent; a different dose of folate is being used in each trial, viz. 0·36 mg daily in the Irish trial (as in Pregnavite forte F) and 4 mg daily in the MRC trial.

What are the Practical Implications? Because the practical implications of this work are, in Smithells' words "enormous and daunting", it is imperative that the efficacy of vitamin supplementation in preventing recurrence of NTD is adequately tested. Hence the need for randomized trials. If these trials show that one or more of the treatments being tested work and should the effect be marked, then it is likely that periconceptional supplementation would be extended to the general childbearing population.

If the efficacy of a vitamin preparation in preventing NTD is shown to be dramatic, one would need to consider a fail-safe method of delivering the efficacious agent to the target population such as fortifying foods. This would apply particularly in countries with a high incidence of these conditions. If it were possible to fortify some very basic foodstuff such as bread with the efficacious agent, this approach has the great advantage of reaching the poorer sections of society where the risk of NTD is highest.

Health education has an important role in attempting to improve the diets of women during their reproductive years. Pre-conception clinics could also be useful but a problem with both health education and pre-conception clinics is that take-up is likely to be poorer among lower social class than among middle class women.

Problems of study design The critical issue in the debate on vitamins and NTD is adequacy of evidence. Because of the problems of study design it is not possible to interpret the findings of Smithells *et al.* (19, 20) in an unbiased manner. Is the effect observed due to the vitamins administered or to the fact that the group of women who selected themselves for supplementation had an inherently low risk of recurrence? The randomized clinical trial is the best methodology available for controlling for such bias.

The history of medicine is replete with examples of regimens that appeared efficacious on the same sort of evidence presented by Smithells and his colleagues until randomized trials demonstrated that they were useless or even harmful (e.g. stilboestrol to prevent spontaneous abortion, clofibrate for the prevention of coronary heart disease, internal mammary ligation for angina, steroids for severe viral hepatitis). Non-randomized clinical trial research designs are much more likely than randomized trials to find therapies beneficial (16). To advocate the widespread implementation of periconceptional vitamin supplementation on the basis of the available evidence and without the support of conclusive randomized trials is, I respectfully suggest, to ignore lessons learned the hard way in medical practice over the past four decades.

1. Antia, A. V., Wiltse, H. E., Rome, R. D., Pitt, E. L., Levin, S., Ottesen, O. E. and Cooke, R. E. (1967). *J. Pediatr.* **71**, 431–41.
2. Averback, P. (1976). Anencephaly associated with megavitamin therapy. *Can. Med. Assoc. J.* **114**, 995.
3. Averback, P. (1976). Anencephaly associated with megavitamin therapy. *Can Med. Assoc. J.* **115**, 725.
4. Bernhardt, I. B. and Dorsey, D. J. (1974). Hypervitaminosis A and congenital renal anomalies in a human infant. *Obstet. Gynecol.* **43**, 750–5.
5. Chalmers, T. C. and Sacks, H. (1982). Vitamin supplements to prevent neural tube defects. *Lancet* **i**, 748.
6. Editorial (1980). Vitamins, neural tube defects and ethics committees. *Lancet* **i**, 1061–2.
7. Friedman, W. F. (1968). Vitamin D and the supravalvular aortic stenosis syndrome. *Adv. Teratol.* **3**, 85–96.
8. Friedman, W. F. and Roberts, W. C. (1966). Vitamin D and the supravalvular aortic stenosis syndrome. *Circulation* **34**, 77–86.
9. Goodenday, L. S. and Gordan, G. S. (1971). No risk from vitamin D in pregnancy. *Ann. Intern. Med.* **75**, 807–8.
10. Laurence, K. M., James, N., Miller, M. H., Tennant, G. B. and Campbell, H. (1981). Double-blind randomized controlled trial of folate treatment before conception to prevent recurrence of neural-tube defects. *Br. Med. J.* **282**, 1509–11.
11. MacCarthy, P. A., Dalrymple, I. J., Duignan, N. M., Elwood, J. H., Guiney, E. J., Hanratty, T. D., Kirke, P. N. and MacDonald, D. W. Recurrence rates of neural tube defects in Dublin maternity hospitals. *Ir. Med. J.* (in press).
12. Meier, P. (1982). Vitamins to prevent neural tube defects. *Lancet* **i**, 859.
13. Nelson, M. M., Forfar, J. (1971). Associations between drugs administered during pregnancy and congenital abnormalities of the fetus. *Br. Med. J.* **i**, 523–7.
14. Nung Won Choi and Klaponski, F. A. (1970). On neural-tube defects: an epidemiological elicitation of etiological factors. *Neurol.* **20**, 399–400.
15. Raab, G. M., Gore, S. M. (1980). Vitamins, neural tube defects and ethics committees. *Lancet* **i**, 1301.
16. Sacks, H., Chalmers, T. C. and Smith, H. (1982). Randomized versus historical controls for clinical trials. *Am. J. Med.* **72**, 233–40.

17. Smithells, R. W. (1982). Prevention of spina bifida: more optimism, less caution. *Link* March/April, pages 8–9.
18. Smithells, R. W., Sheppard, S., Schorah, C. J., Seller, M. J., Nevin, N. C., Harris, R., Read, A. P. and Fielding, D. W. (1980) Possible prevention of neural tube defects by periconceptional vitamin supplementation. *Lancet* i, 339–40.
19. Smithells, R. W., Sheppard, S., Schorah, C. J., Seller, M. J., Nevin, N. C., Harris, R., Read, A. P., Fielding, D. W. and Walker, S. (1981). Vitamin supplementation and neural tube defects. *Lancet* ii, 1425.
20. Smithells, R. W., Sheppard, S., Schorah, C. J., Seller, M. J., Nevin, N. C., Harris, R., Read, A. P. and Fielding, D. W. (1981). Apparent prevention of neural tube defects by periconceptional vitamin supplementation. *Arch. Dis. Child.* 56, 911–18.
21. Stone, D. H. (1980). Possible prevention of neural tube defects by periconceptional vitamin supplementation. *Lancet* i, 647.

Author's reply: The difference in social class distribution between fully supplemented and unsupplemented women is acknowledged (but see "Matching for Social Class" later). The difference in previous obstetric history is more apparent than real, a point fully discussed in our *Arch. Dis. Child.* Dec. 1981 paper (Chapter 3, ref. 13).

Has Kirke misunderstood the numbers of women withdrawn or excluded (1, 2)? *Two* women were excluded. The others either withdrew before becoming pregnant or were not pregnant when the first cohort was closed and were transferred to the 2nd cohort.

Very few withdrew themselves after agreeing to supplementation. These few were in N. Ireland and Nevin confirms that they were *not* transferred to the "unsupplemented" group. (However, had they been transferred, the analogy with Laurence's transfer of non-compliant "folate" mothers to the placebo group is of doubtful validity.)

The fascinating observation that the National Maternity and the Coombe Hospitals have such strikingly different recurrence rates (though the National "rate" derives from a single case) prompts me to ask two questions:

(1) How are patients distributed between the two hospitals? The Coombe is as far above the Dublin mean as the National is below.
(2) What are the prenatal vitamin supplementation policies at these two hospitals? Folate supplements to the end of pregnancy affect folate levels 3 months later and are therefore preconceptional if the next conception is not much delayed (Schorah *et al.*, in press).

Dr Kirke does not feel secure about the safety of vitamin supplements and suggests following several thousand babies into childhood, but offers no evidence to support his fears. The two studies he cites (13, 14) give no data on administration of iron and vitamins *before the sixth week* of pregnancy.

Iron cannot be absorbed in excess. However, the composition of an "ideal" vitamin supplement is certainly open to discussion.

As regards mothers taking excessive doses, this is a risk with *any* drug prescribed or purchased and is not normally regarded as a reason to withhold it. Laurence calculates that a woman would have to take 200 tablets of Pregnavite forte F at one fell swoop to achieve an amount of vitamin A that would begin to worry him. It is not *our* practice to issue such quantities at any one time. The risk of folic acid masking pernicious anaemia in women of child-bearing age is very much smaller than the risk of megaloblastic anaemia of pregnancy.

1. Chalmers, T. C. and Sacks, H. (1982). Vitamin supplements to prevent neural tube defects. *Lancet* **i**, 748.
2. Smithells, R. W., Sheppard, S., Schorah, C. J., Seller, M. J., Nevin, N. C., Harris, R., Read, A. P. and Fielding, D. W. (1982). Vitamin supplements and neural tube defects. *Lancet* **i**, 1186.

Paedar Kirke's reply: In relation to the marked difference in the recurrence rate between the Coombe and the National Maternity hospitals Professor Smithells asked about the social class distributions of the mothers attending these hospitals and he also sought information on the prenatal vitamin supplementation policies at the hospitals.

An examination of the social class profiles of the Dublin maternity hospitals carried out in 1979 (Kirke, unpublished data) showed that the National Maternity had a higher proportion of mothers in the upper social classes than the Coombe but the hospital difference was not very marked.

I discussed the prenatal vitamin supplementation policies at the two hospitals during the period 1970–6 with Dr Clinch who was Master at the Coombe during 1971–7 and with Dr Meagher, Master at the National Maternity during 1970–6. In both hospitals all mothers were prescribed Folferite [R] (compound ferrous sulphate 193 mg and folic acid 0·5 mg per tablet (Glaxo)) in a dosage of one tablet twice daily from the time of booking until the end of the first week after delivery. In the Coombe hospital a small proportion of private patients may have been prescribed alternative iron-folate preparations (e.g. Fefol [R]). The hospitals had a different supplementation policy following discharge. In the Coombe hospital only those mothers who were clinically anaemic (incidence 7% in 1970–6) were supplemented; they were continued on the same iron-folate preparation until their anaemia responded. In the National Maternity hospital all mothers were given a container of 100 Folferite tablets at discharge and were advised to take one tablet twice daily until the tablets were finished. Neither Dr Clinch nor Dr Meagher felt that they could make a realistic estimate of the proportion of mothers delivering in their hospitals in 1970–5 who would become pregnant again within the following 3 to 6 months. It would be possible, although time-consuming, to examine the pregnancy intervals for the mothers in the study (1). I would prefer first to repeat the recurrence study for the mothers who had affected babies in the study hospitals during 1976–80 to see if the hospital differences in recurrence noted in the first cohort (1) are similar for the 1976–80 cohort.

1. MacCarthy, P. A., Dalrymple, I. J., Duignan, N. M., Elwood, J. H., Guiney, E. J., Hanratty, T. D., Kirke, P. N., MacDonald, D. W. Recurrence rates of neural tube defects in Dublin maternity hospitals. *Ir. Med. J.* (in press).

Michael Laurence: This is an excellent well-balanced succinct account of prevention of neural tube defects by vitamin supplementation and also of the role of diet. Professor Smithells posed some specific questions regarding the prevention studies by Laurence *et al.*

The Methods of Assessing Maternal Diet. It is agreed that when trying to assess the total intake of the different dietary constituents, the only reliable methods to hand are those of 24 h recall and of the weighing method extended over several days, preferably a week, which would require careful supervision. Neither method would have been satisfactory for our purposes or our subjects. The former was judged to give too narrow a picture and the latter was thought to be inappropriate as our patients were unlikely to have been suitable for the weighing method even with considerable supervision as they would have been not really capable of carrying it through, and we suspected that they would have modified their diet during the period of study. As we were largely interested in folic acid containing foods it was felt that we would be able to obtain sufficient information from a check list of the pattern of meals that our subjects were taking. The retrospective assessment of diet taken during the first trimester of pregnancy sometimes as long as 10–15 years previously may well have been both biased and faulty. Although this part of the study was reported, it was not the main part of the investigation. However, the responses were remarkably consistent. The diet that women took in the normal non pregnant state was based on the diet taken immediately previous to the interviewer's visit and in most instances according to the mother's report, seemed usually to vary remarkably little from week to week. The diet recorded "prospectively" during the first trimester of the prospectively studied pregnancies was that taken during the previous week or so and was indeed assessed by the interviewer at the time of the interview or just after but was then re-assessed by a research assistant using a scoring method. There was almost 100% agreement between the two assessments. The former was obviously done without knowledge of the outcome of the prospectively studied pregnancies, the latter did have access to the information about outcome of pregnancy.

Some patients in the dietary counselling study did also receive folate supplementation, others received placebo, a considerable proportion had neither. Folate supplementation was likely to have reduced the dietary effects, therefore, had no supplementation been given the results might have been more striking. Although the effect of dietary counselling would not be influenced materially one, possibly two, additional patients on a poor diet might have had a recurrence. The study was originally one to investigate the biochemical aspects of early pregnancy in women at increased risk and of the effect of folic acid supplementation. The dietary study was added after the pilot study as it was felt that this was an essential background investigation for the former.

Dietary habits of women are largely determined by their early upbringing and influences during childhood and their own feeding habits, likes and dislikes tend to remain remarkably resistant to dietary counselling. My co-workers tell me that a considerable proportion of mothers on a poor diet provide much more satisfactory meals for both husband and the children. Dietary counselling seems to have been quite effective for these women who were anxious to avoid recurrence and were therefore well motivated. However, in many instances, once pregnancy was over they reverted at least partially towards their former dietary habits.

In answer to Professor Smithell's specific query, folic acid supplementation begun once contraceptive measures were stopped was continued until the end of the first trimester.

The serum folate is influenced by a number of ephemeral factors such as the content of recent meals and the time since the last meal. It represents largely transport folate and would therefore not be expected to be as closely related to such factors as social class and quality of the normal diet. Vitamin B_{12}, referred to by Professor Smithells, was also measured in our study and I hope to have information on B_{12} levels on our patients available for the October meeting. My impression at present is that there was a much more ephemeral relationship between diet and B_{12} levels than between diet and red cell folate and that in those pregnancies ending in anencephalics, the B_{12} level in first trimester was not particularly depressed.

The study by Hibbard and Smithells (see Chapter 3, ref. 4) in Liverpool seems to show that folic acid supplementation during early pregnancy (but not preconceptionally given) reduces the abortion risk. Our dietary study also seems to suggest that a better diet reduces the risk.

Do Vitamin Supplements do any Harm? Some women who have been recommended to have preconceptional supplementation have in fact planned to have this to prevent a recurrence, finding themselves pregnant sooner than planned might well panic and attempt to make up for not taking the tablets soon enough take large quantities at once, as several patients in our investigation have done, including one of the "non-compliers". Under such circumstances a woman might possibly take a potentially teratogenic dose of vitamin A or a harmful amount of vitamin D.

The high (quite unphysiological) amount of folic acid in our study was prescribed in order to overcome any absorption defect or partial metabolic block of folic acid. We were not aware of any folic acid intolerance and do not think that the high dose contributed to the high non-compliance rate. High non-compliance is apparently quite common in pregnancy.

Decline in Incidence and Recurrence In no family studies reported is there a suggestion that a drop in the incidence is accompanied by an equal drop in the risk of recurrence. The latter is usually much less marked.

What is the Mechanism of Action? Any one of the three mechanisms for folic acid unavailability to the fetus or a combination of them may be at fault in an individual case. Certainly folic acid deficiency as such must be rare but there seems to be some suggestion that excessive amounts of carbohydrates impair the absorption of dietary folic acid.

Polyglutamate Absorption Test The possibility of a polyglutamate absorption test is an interesting one. It might identify women who have low folic acid stores in women who are known to be at increased risk but it would seem hardly to be the sort of test that can be applied on a population basis to identify those women potentially at risk who have not got any family or obstetric history of NTD.

Preconception Clinics Preconception clinics are an obvious development in obstetrics to achieve improvements in maternal health before pregnancy is begun and prevention of neural tube defects by maternal diet improvement in those at increased risk by supplementation. It may well not be very successful in the former.

Problems of Study Design In the proposed MRC study it may well not be possible to use placebo containing no vitamins as had been proposed. This will not necessarily negate the study but it might well lead to its prolongation.

Editor's note: See also comments on Smithells' paper in Appendix III.

The Role of Improvement in the Maternal Diet and Preconceptional Folic Acid Supplementation in the Prevention of Neural Tube Defects

K. M. LAURENCE

Department of Child Health,
Welsh National School of Medicine, Cardiff

H. CAMPBELL

Welsh National School of Medicine, Cardiff

NANSI E. JAMES*

Department of Child Health,
Welsh National School of Medicine, Cardiff

Introduction

The neural tube defects (NTD) which include anencephaly, encephalocoele, myelocoele (myelomeningocoele), meningocoele and complicated spina bifida occulta but not isolated hydrocephalus or simple spina bifida occulta, are different end products of the same general process and are now widely accepted to have a multifactorial aetiology (4). A major genetic component which is thought to be polygenic, renders the embryo susceptible to interference during the fourth week after conception by intrauterine environmental factors. There are likely to be a number of such factors, perhaps with different ones being of major importance in various populations with a high

* Not present at the Workshop.

incidence. As there is very little likelihood of being able effectively to modify the genetic component, primary prevention of the NTDs would therefore be dependent on being able to identify the environmental trigger factors so that they can either be removed from the environment or be avoided. However, although NTDs can be produced in experimental animals by numerous and very differing environmental insults, intensive epidemiological and clinical studies in man have only recently produced evidence of a specific environmental factor which might be of aetiological importance, poor maternal nutrition and more specifically, folic acid depletion and folate antagonists.

Maternal nutrition has been suspected as an aetiological factor for some time because in the British Isles with its high incidence, those regions that seem to be more deprived such as the Irish Republic, Northern Ireland, South Wales, the North West of England, and the South West of Scotland have the highest incidence. Within these areas and elsewhere social class IV and V families have a much higher incidence than those of social class I and II (15, 20, 23). There has been a seasonal variation as well, with a higher prevalence amongst conceptions in winter and spring when fresh foods are less plentiful and more expensive (15). In the last decade or so, not only has the general incidence of NTD fallen dramatically in the United Kingdom (2), especially in the high incidence regions (12, 21), but also social class differences and seasonal variations have been less pronounced (15). These changes may be due to the improvement in the general standard of maternal nutrition and could in part be due to the more widespread use of imported fresh vegetables available throughout the year and the increased use of "fresh" deep frozen food. Another explanation might be the greater use of family planning in lower social class couples (11). Secular trends have been noted in the past and have usually been difficult to interpret. However, the sharp rise in the incidence of NTD in Boston during the depression years (19) has been interpreted as being due to poor maternal nutrition prevailing at the time.

Studies in South Wales

To elucidate these problems further we carried out various studies in South Wales into the nutritional status of women who had had conceptions with a neural tube defect and we have completed a trial of supplementation of the pre- and post-conceptional diet before and during the first trimester of subsequent pregnancies by these women.

First Dietary Study

In this study we identified women living in the Counties of Glamorgan and Gwent who had had a child with a neural tube defect between 1954 and 1974. This was a population in which there had been several epidemiologic studies and several registers of patients were available. Those who were still under 35 years of age were visited between 1969 and 1974 (17) by two investigators. Both investigators were doctors, one with a long experience of taking dietary histories in diabetic clinics and the other with wide experience in public health clinics and general practice. One surveyed the western half of the area, and the other the eastern areas.

Nine hundred and two women were visited in their homes; 442 women who were not pregnant and who had not decided to have any more children were enrolled in the dietary study.

The women in the dietary study were interrogated about their usual diet at the time of the survey, this was called the interpregnancy diet. Enquiries concerning diet in previous pregnancies were made, but these do not form part of this report.

A simple diet sheet was used that provided a general pattern for meals and a check list (see Appendix 1) which included protein-rich foods, dairy products, vegetables and fruits, brown and white bread, confectionery and soft drinks, and was designed to reveal any deficiency in the consumption of foods containing significant amounts of folic acid during an average week.

The diets were classified as "good", "fair" or "poor". Good diets were those comprising a large variety of foods including particularly meats, eggs and milk, green vegetables and fruit, and with a relatively low consumption of confectionery and soft drinks. Such a diet would be expected to provide generous intakes of all the nutrients (including folic acid) and dietary fibre. Poor diets were monotonous, restricted in variety, with very low intakes of animal foods, including milk, and of fruits and vegetables, and an over-dependence on "convenience foods" high in carbohydrate and fat. These diets were often associated with irregular meal patterns, and a high consumption of confectionery, and would provide marginal intakes of vitamins and minerals. The diets judged to be "fair" were intermediate between these extremes, but in addition were thought to provide low intakes of one or more nutrients. This classification was carried out by an independent research worker after the end of the study who was unaware of the outcome of pregnancies. This reassessment was re-examined by one of us (NJ) but almost no changes to the independent classification were made at this stage.

Blood samples were taken after the interview, but conditions under which they were taken (as to time of month and day, and relationship to meals) could not be standardized. Serum and red cell folic acid concentrations were measured and vitamin B_{12} was also measured (9, 35). Haematocrit was also estimated.

The women in the western area of Glamorgan who were willing to co-operate in the prospective study were counselled to improve their diets and to stop smoking not later than the time when contraceptive precautions were stopped. Those in the eastern area were not specifically counselled. Both groups were instructed to report to us within 6 weeks of the last menstrual period if they missed a period. They were revisited as soon as possible and certainly before the 11th week from the LMP and detailed enquiries were made about the quality of the diet during the pregnancy so far, about illness, nausea and vomiting and medicines used. Another blood sample was taken and the same haematological and biochemical factors measured. They were revisited at least twice more, in mid-pregnancy and immediately after the end of the pregnancy.

Results of First Dietary Study

There were 442 who were eligible for admission to this study. Of these 26 subsequently proved to be pregnant at interview and one was on folate treatment leaving 415 subjects in the study. Of these only 65 reported a good interpregnancy diet, 197 a fair diet and 149 a poor diet; four diet histories could not be analysed. The mean serum folate concentration and the red cell folate for these groups are shown in Table 1 and the gradient of the measurements suggests that the dietary assessment had some validity. Serum B_{12} concentration did not correlate with this classification of diet.

Table 1. First Dietary Study.

Women with a previous fetal neural tube defect. Quality of interpregnancy diet and mean concentration of serum folate red blood cell folate and serum B_{12}.

Quality of diet	Subjects n	%	Mean serum folate μg/l	RBC folate μg/l of red cells	Serum B_{12} μg/l
Good	65	16	8·9	295	283
Fair	197	47	5·4	236	272
Poor	149	36	4·9	197	285[a]
Not known	4	1			
All women	415	100	5·9	238	277

[a] Two sera with concentrations of B_{12} over 1000 μg/l excluded as subjects were likely to have been on B_{12} treatment.

Of these 415 women, 174 reported within adequate time, 186 subsequent confirmed pregnancies, of whom 12 reported twice. They were all revisited within 11 weeks of their last menstrual period, a current pregnancy dietary history taken and a blood sample taken. There were 103 from West Glamorgan and 71 from East Glamorgan or Gwent.

In previous epidemiological studies we had found no obvious differences in the social and demographic characteristics of the women in the two areas (15) and their diets in the interpregnancy period and during the first trimester of previous pregnancies were similar.

In the western area where all women had been counselled to improve their diet the majority had heeded this advice and almost three quarters (71%) had improved their diet in time for their next pregnancy and the reason why many of the remainder did not do so was because of excessive nausea and vomiting (Table 2). In the uncounselled area over 80% did not change the pattern of their diet. The outcome of the 109 pregnancies in the western area

Table 2. First Dietary Study.

Change in diet in Project Pregnancy compared to that in Index Pregnancy.

Instructions on diet	Improved		Change in Diet No change		Worse		All pregnancies
	n	%	n	%	n	%	n
Counselled	78	71	29	27	2	2	109
Not counselled	9	12	63	82	5	6	77
All diets	87	47	92	49	7	4	186

[a] Six counselled women and 6 non-counselled women had two pregnancies. [b] The project pregnancy diet was recorded at the time of this pregnancy. [c] The index pregnancy diet was taken by recall at the interpregnancy interview.

was 10 miscarriages and three recurrences of neural tube defects; amongst the 77 in the eastern area there were eight miscarriages and five recurrences. The ratio of the risk of recurrence in east Glamorgan compared to west Glamorgan was 2·4 although this did not differ statistically significantly from 1·0.

Table 3 shows the pattern of recurrence of NTD and of miscarriages in these 186 pregnancies. All eight recurrences occurred in women whose diets were considered to be poor during the first trimester of that pregnancy, an assessment which was made at the time of the first visit during the pregnancy before any outcome could be known. There were no recurrences in the pregnancies with a good or fair diet. This distribution was most unlikely to have occurred by chance ($P<0·001$).

K. M. Laurence et al.

Table 3. First Dietary Study.

Outcome of Project Pregnancies. By Quality of Diet in First Trimester.

Outcome of pregnancy	Good n	Quality of diet Fair n	Poor n	All pregnancies n
Normal child	53	85	22	160
Recurrent NTD	–	–	8	8
Miscarriage	–	3	15	18
All outcomes	53	88	45	186

It should also be noted that 15 miscarriages occurred to 45 women with poor diets whereas only three occurred in the 141 pregnancies with moderate or good diets. Of the three women with recurrences who had received counselling, one had ignored the advice but two suffered nausea and vomiting during the first month of conception which had continued into hyperemesis gravidarum.

Second Dietary Study

A second dietary study was conducted between 1974 and 1979 largely in West Glamorgan, again with women who had at least one previous pregnancy with an NTD, but this time two control groups were also studied; the sisters of these who have had only normal babies and a group of University and professional wives (10). The dietary investigation was based on a modified form of Burke's dietary history which was more detailed than the one used in the first study (3). The diet was again divided into three main categories of good, fair and poor; we included within the poor diets those subjects whose diet would have been considered to have been fair except that it was unbalanced by excessive amounts of refined carbohydrates and fats.

The 244 index women visited in their homes were found to have a dietary pattern very similar to the women in the previous dietary study. One hundred out of 244 (41%) seemed to be on a poor diet. This compared with 32 out of 123 (26%) amongst their sister controls, and 3 out of 50 (6%) of the upper class controls (Table 4). All the women in this study were given dietary counselling with apparently even greater effect than in the previous study. The 244 "index women" had 176 further pregnancies by the end of 1979 during which only 32 (18%) remained on a poor diet. These 176 preg-

Table 4. Secondary Dietary Study.

Interpregnancy Diet. Cases and Controls. Number of subjects and row percent.

| | Quality of diet | | | | | | | | All |
| | Good | | Fair | | Poor (a) | | Poor (b) | | All |
Group of women	n	%	n	%	n	%	n	%	cases
Index cases	34	14	110	45	33	14	67	27	244
Sisters controls	43	35	48	39	23	19	9	7	123
Upper class controls	39	78	8	16	3	6	0	0	50

[a] All diets were current interpregnancy diets. [b] Index cases had had a pregnancy with a fetal NTD. [c] Sisters of index cases who had not had a NTD. [d] Upper class controls, university and professional wives who had not had a NTD. [e] Poor diets are subdivided into (a) those with an adequate diet but excess refined carbohydrates and fat, (b) those with a totally inadequate diet.

nancies resulted in 5 NTDs (2·8%) which is about half the number of recurrences expected. But more important, all five recurrences occurred in the 32 pregnancies with disordered diets, a rate of 16%. This distribution was unlikely to have occurred by chance ($P<0·01$) (Table 5).

Table 5. Secondary Dietary Study.

Diet of Index women during first trimester of project pregnancy.

| | Quality of diet | | | | | | | | All |
| Outcome | Good | | Fair | | Poor (a) | | Poor (b) | | pregnancies |
to fetus	n	%	n	%	n	%	n	%	n
Normal	68	40	76	44	15	9	12	7	171
NTD					3	60	2	40	5
All fetuses	68	39	76	43	18	10	14	8	176

[a] Seven index women had had two previous pregnancies with NTD. [b] 176 index women became pregnant and 5 had a NTD giving a rate of 2·8%. All recurrences had poor diets. [c] All women were counselled to improve their diet.

Folate Deficiency as a Possible Cause of NTD

Although the effect of poor maternal nutrition on the developing embryo may be due to a number of vitamin deficiencies acting together to interfere with the closure of the neural tube, or may allow some as yet unidentified teratogen to have an influence (24), it seemed to us much more likely that the main cause, in the British Isles at least, was a lack of folate, basing our judgement on evidence that was experimental, embryological, epidemiological as well as clinical.

NTD can be induced in the rat by exposing developing embryos to a variety of teratogens (7b) including anti-folic acid agents after the 9th day following fertilization. In the rat the neural tube begins to form about the 8th or 9th day, closure being complete towards the middle of the 12th day (1). This is also the stage when in the rat embryo, the chorio-allantoic placenta begins to develop and the embryonic heart starts to perfuse it and the pace of the development and energy requirement increases significantly (1). During this time there are also considerable changes in the metabolic processes. Before the neural tube is formed the rat embryo largely derives its energy from glycolysis and the pentose phosphate shunt, but from that time there is a progressive switch to the Krebs cycle (26, 34). In the chick embryo it seems to have been shown that neural tube closure is critically dependent on an oxygen gradient in the neural crests (38), producing only a narrow band of hypoxic surface cells along the opposing neural crests. Lack of sufficient folate at that stage or a general metabolic disturbance, could then interfere with the normal closure process and either the crests do not meet correctly or if they do meet the hypoxic necrosis has progressed too far and so they dehisce again.

It may be thought that these findings in rodent or bird embryo bear little relation to the situation in man. However, "it is an accepted principle of comparative embryology that species differences in form and structure become less striking as earlier embryonic stages are examined and it is an interesting, but largely unstudied possibility that inter-species metabolic differences are also minimal in the early embryo" (39).

Translated to the human embryo, all these processes take place between the 21st and 25th day after fertilization, and there is every reason to suppose that they differ only in detail and in timing from those in the chick and the rat. It is not possible to investigate the metabolic processes in human embryos at that stage of development.

However, further research using the technique of New (22), should be able to throw light on the precise changes in folate requirements and the influence that the various micronutrients, etc. have on development. This may give some indication of the role that they play in early human development. We found that both the serum and the red cell folate levels are low in women who are on an unsatisfactory diet (Table 1), and Smithells found similar results in women from social class III, IV and V, both when not pregnant and during the first trimester (27; and see page 197), but especially so at the beginning of a pregnancy that ended in an infant with an NTD (28). Finally there is the small human experience with aminopterin in precipitating NTD (36).

Folic Acid Supplementation Trial

A double blind randomized controlled trial of folate treatment compared to an inert placebo given before conception and continuing until at least the 12th week of pregnancy was started in South Wales in 1969 and continued until 1974 (14, 18). The subjects were recruited from the same women who at the same time were taking part in the first dietary study. On recruitment to that study, all these women were asked if they would be prepared to take part in a study of the possible causes of NTD, and as part of this they were invited to take tablets at the beginning of their next pregnancy, without any promise of success. Those who agreed to take part were randomized to two treatment groups, either 2 mg twice a day of folic acid in the form of methyl folate in an inert tablet, or the identical tablet of inert filler without folic acid. They were told to advise the investigators as soon as they intended to stop contraceptive precautions; tablets were then sent to them which they were instructed to take until they missed a period when they were to notify the field workers as soon as possible when they were sensitized by the field workers. Treatment was continued up to 12 weeks of pregnancy. Women

Table 6. Folic Acid Supplementation Trial.

Recurrence of Neural Tube Defects.

| Case | Treatment | Diet | Wk. | Blood Estimations | | | Outcome | | |
				Serum Folate	Red Cell Folate	B_{12}	Delivery	Lesion	Gestation Mths.
A	F.NC	Poor	7	212·0	259	112	MC	AN	3
B	F.NC	Poor	8	4·8	155	167	LB	SB	9
C	PL	Poor	8	3·7	228	89	LB	SB	8
D	PL	Poor	7	11·0	275	210	MC	AN	4
E	PL	Poor	8	5·0	380	217	LB	SB	9
F	PL	Poor	7	2·9	76	371	T	AN	5

Estimations in μg/l. F.NC = Folate Non-complier. PL = Placebo. LB = Live birth.
MC = Miscarriage. AN = Anencephalic. SB = Spina bifida cystica.
Case A. Past history: 1 surviving spina bifida, 1 miscarriage. Diet known to be poor, excessive carbohydrate intake. Took no tablets until 7 weeks after LMP. She then took a considerable number 24 hours before blood sample was taken and then continued to take the tablets as instructed. We did not know this until after the end of the whole trial. Outcome, anencephalic miscarriage at 12 weeks.
Case B. Past history: 2 normal children, 2 anencephalics and 4 spontaneous abortions. Diet very poor. Started to take tablets 7–10 days after LMP at a time when she was feeling sick, off work with febrile illness. The nausea increased to vomiting and she returned most of the tablets she was taking. Her diet up to 8/52 after LMP was largely milk. Thereafter she felt much better. Outcome full term spina bifida female, died on first day.

who did not apply for tablets or who received tablets but did not report back that they had become pregnant were not revisited at this stage.

Neither the doctor nor the subject knew the treatment allocated so that this would not influence their willingness to take the tablets, their response to notifying a suspect pregnancy nor the field workers' thoroughness in making the recall visit and taking a history. Once the history had been taken and a blood sample analysed and the pregnancy confirmed there was no point in maintaining the anonymity of the treatment as the outcome could not be subject to any form of subjective bias, although in practice the code was not broken at this time.

Results of Intervention Trial

All the women who were approached in connection with the first dietary study and folate trial are analysed in Appendix II. There were 415 women who were not pregnant nor on folate therapy in the dietary study. Of these 197 were unwilling to take part in a trial of an unspecified treatment with no assurance of success but were willing to help with the dietary follow-up. Two hundred and eighteen were willing to take part in a trial. Of these 114 were allocated at random to folate treatment and 104 to placebo. Appendix II gives a complete schedule of the various groups into which the 442 women were analysed.

The criteria for entry to the folate analysis group were more stringent than those for the dietary study. They had to be seen within 11 weeks of last menstrual period, they had to provide a pregnancy dietary history, the serum folate concentration had to be reported by the laboratory. There were 123 pregnancies reported which met these criteria, 60 in the folate group and 63 in the placebo group.

Analysis of Compliance

As it is well known that patients and especially pregnant women do not necessarily take medicines prescribed we used the serum folate concentration as a screening test. When we came to the analyses we decided that if the folate subjects had a serum level below 10 μg/l they would be considered as non-compliers. There were 15 subjects classified as non-compliers by this criterion. Similar results would have been obtained if we had used red cell folate at a level of 350 μg/l of red cells. The detailed distributions of serum folate and red cell folate are shown in Figs 1(a) and 1(b). We had no test of compliance in the placebo group. We had not asked the subjects to confirm

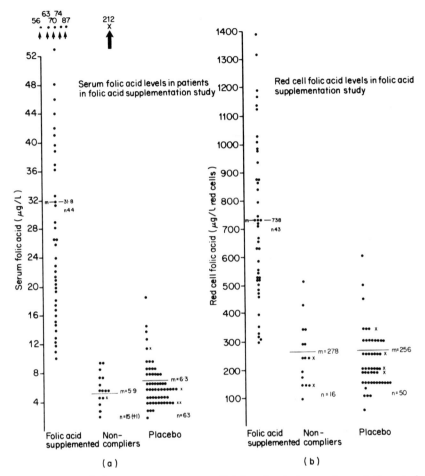

Fig. 1. (a) and (b). Serum and red cell folate levels in supplementation study divided into groups according to whether the patients were on folic acid supplementation or placebo, or whether they were non-compliers. All but one of those regarded to have been non-compliers had serum folate levels below 10 mg/l. (x denotes patients with a recurrence.)

that they had taken the tablets in the early years of the study, but in later years we were able to confirm in some cases that there was non-compliance. While it is reasonable to infer that there was non-compliance from the low folate levels, the possibility that poor absorption may be a cause of low serum folate in some individuals could not be excluded.

We were surprised to find one woman in the folate tablet group with a serum folate level of 212 μg/l with a low red cell folate 259 μg/l, but we

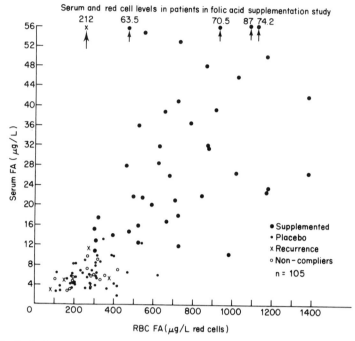

Fig. 2. Relationship between red and serum folate levels. All those on folic acid supplementation had greatly elevated serum and red cell folate levels. (X = recurrence; O = non-compliers; ● = placebo; ● = folate supplemented).

considered this possibly a laboratory error of estimation and we retained her as a folate complier. She had a miscarriage of an anencephalic fetus at 12 weeks of pregnancy. We have the specimen. In 1980 at the time of the publicity following the publication of the paper by Smithells et al. (29) she came to one of us and admitted that she had not taken the tablets during early pregnancy but when she realized that the field worker would take a blood sample she swallowed a large number on the evening before the visit. We examined a cross tabulation of serum folate against red cell folate (Fig. 2) and found a reasonable degree of association except for this one subject who had a low red cell concentration yet this extraordinarily high serum concentration. Her diet before pregnancy and during pregnancy had been poor, her B_{12} concentration was consonant with the poor dietary history (112 $\mu g/l$). We accepted her story and reclassified her as a non-complier.

The outcome of these pregnancies are shown in Tables 6, 7 and 8. There were four recurrences out of 63 (6·4%) in the placebo group and two recurrences out of 60 (3·3%) in the folate prescribed group. Although the relative risk was 2·0 or a possible 50% reduction in recurrences this could

Table 7. Folic Acid Supplementation Trial.

Outcome of Pregnancy by Treatment Group.

Outcome of pregnancy	Folate supplement Compliers	Folate supplement Non-compliers	Placebo supplement	All cases
Normal fetus	44	14	59	117
Neural tube defect	0	2	4	6
All outcomes	44	16	63	123

not be considered significant statistically as the numbers were so small. However, it is important to note that the two recurrent cases in the folate prescribed group were both non-compliers and so six recurrences occurred in 79 unsupplemented pregnancies ($7 \cdot 6\%$) and none in the 44 supplemented pregnancies (Fisher's exact test $P = 0 \cdot 04$). Thus the data suggest that there was a biological effect of folate which could be demonstrated even though in practice it was difficult to ensure that women took the tablets and so achieve satisfactory results. The specific effect of taking folate had to be separated from the more general effect of diet. There were no recurrences among 91 pregnancies who received good or fair diets but there were six recurrences amongst the 32 pregnancies receiving a poor diet ($P<0 \cdot 001$ Fisher's exact test) (Table 8). Within this high risk group of women, however, there were no recurrences in the 10 who had taken folate supplementation but six in the 22 who had poor diet and had not taken supplementation ($P = 0 \cdot 004$ Fisher's exact test). Thus, although there may have been some bias owing to women who were receiving an inadequate diet also failing to comply, within this group receiving an inadequate diet the preventive effect of supplementation despite an inadequate diet could still be detected.

Table 8. Folic Acid Supplement Trial.

Outcome of Pregnancy by Quality of Diet in First Trimester; by Folate Supplementation Received.

Outcome of pregnancy	Good F	Good NF	Fair F	Fair NF	Poor F	Poor NF	All Diets F	All Diets NF
Normal fetus	18	25	16	32	10	16	44	73
Neural tube defect	0	0	0	0	0	6	0	6
All outcomes	18	25	16	32	10	22	44	79

F = Folate supplemented.   NF = Folate not supplemented.

Other Pregnancies Resulting in Neural Tube Defects

We are aware of seven further pregnancies which resulted in a fetus with a NTD occurring amongst the women in these studies which are listed in Appendix III. Four of these pregnancies were excluded because they were not visited within the prescribed 11 weeks from LMP. This was because these women had not requested tablets before conception or notified the pregnancy to us within the 11 weeks. Two patients had been in group 0 who had refused to take tablets, one had been randomized to the A group (folate) and one to the B group (placebo). Three other pregnancies occurred after the close of the trial, two from the B group and one from the A group. These pregnancies were unsupplemented as no tablets were sent to them.

All seven of these patients had poor pregnancy diets and one of them had had a previous normal pregnancy in the dietary study when she took no tablets, but improved her diet. In the subsequent pregnancy outside the study period she relapsed to a poor diet, took no tablets and had a fetus with spina bifida systica mildly affected who survived.

These further cases confirm our trial conclusions that a poor diet greatly increases the risk of a neural tube defect and offer no evidence either way on the efficiency of folate therapy.

Discussion

This supplementation study seems to demonstrate that folic acid unavailability to the embryo during the first 4 weeks of development is an important aetiological factor in NTDs in South Wales at least, and probably in the British Isles in general, and that dietary supplementation seems to prevent recurrences (32, 33, 34). It also suggests that the folic acid content of Pregnavite forte F, used in the highly successful supplementation trial of Smithells and his colleagues, is the major if not the only active substance (21). It is not necessary that diets in the first trimester of women who have a fetus with an NTD need always be frankly deficient in foods containing folic acid. Much of the folic acid content of food is often destroyed, first in storage, in processing (e.g. canning), and then in the preparation of the meals. Some women cannot take their usual diet as they suffer from nausea and vomiting almost from the time that they conceive. Analogous to the absorption of dietary zinc (28), that of folates may be interfered with by excessive amounts of refined carbohydrates and fats which are so common in the diet of women in South Wales. In others a disordered metabolism of folic acid may also play a part for there seems to be a suggestion that a greater proportion of women who have just had a child with an NTD show evidence of impaired folic acid metabolism than do women with a normal outcome (8).

Conclusion

What we had demonstrated therefore was that in the circumstances of South Wales in 1969–74 it was very difficult to establish a trial of preventive treatment in pregnancy and there was no assurance that the subjects would actually comply with a protocol, but that if the serum folate level and the red cell folate could be raised above critical thresholds then there were no recurrences of neural tube defects in a high risk group of women.

The two dietary studies were based upon a pragmatic classification of the quality of the diets, but the detailed histories on which they were based were extensive and had been taken by two clinical field workers widely experienced in taking dietary histories from women in these population groups.

They demonstrate first that women who have had a fetal neural tube defect were more likely than others to be taking a poor diet; in the first study there was no control group for comparison purposes, but in our second study there were two comparison groups, the sisters of the index cases and the wives of professional families in the same area. The current diets of the index cases were markedly poorer than those of either control group.

They demonstrate secondly, that it is possible to persuade women to change their diet and three-quarters of the counselled group had made considerable improvements compared to only about a tenth of the group not counselled.

They demonstrate thirdly, that in the prospective survey all the recurrences occurred in the group of women who were shown to have a poor diet from the history taken contemporaneously at the second month of pregnancy.

The supplementation trial demonstrates first that such trials are very difficult to undertake. We offered no assurances, placed no pressure on the women to join the trial, avoided publicity and did not follow up those women who did not return voluntarily to the field workers. This reduced our possible population by three-quarters. Now that assurances can be given and publicity cannot be avoided the response should be much better.

Secondly, there is a serious problem of how to ensure that any treatment has been taken and how this can be validated. Probably a quarter of the women who did return to us were not taking the medications.

Thirdly, it is essential to distinguish between the effectiveness of an agent which has been used in preventing recurrences and the efficiency of a regime in converting an effective agent into a usable efficient system of treatment. The trial demonstrated that no recurrences occurred to women who took the folate, whether or not they had an adequate diet; similarly no recurrences occurred to women who had an adequate diet whether or not they were supplemented; all the recurrences occurred in the small group who had poor diets and were not supplemented.

The trial, therefore, is persuasive that neural tube defects are the result of deficient diet and that they can be prevented either by an adequate diet or by supplementation with folate. It does not exclude the possibility that there are other deficiencies or some abnormality of folic acid metabolism (8) which can be swamped by an excessive intake of folate.

Contrary to what has been suggested recently (6) we do not consider that the time has come for supplementation to be used on a population scale or if it were that it would be efficient. A well controlled study improving on the defects of the previous studies is still required (5). Our trial was too small and was confined to a particular group within a particular ethnic group for extrapolation to be made with confidence and the Pregnavite forte F trial was defective because of the choice of controls (7a, 25, 29, 33). We therefore support the proposal for a large multi-centred randomized controlled trial to prevent recurrence of neural tube defects.

With the prospect of effective preconceptional supplementation to prevent NTD, improvement in the general diet and especially in the maternal diet before conception must not be overlooked. Effective dietary education of our mothers-to-be should become an essential part of the school curriculum and every effort should be made to continue this process after leaving school (17). In addition, any woman who has had a pregnancy resulting in NTD or is at increased risk because of a strong family history should be given dietary counselling before embarking on a pregnancy. Dietary counselling for motivated women, if carried out sympathetically and authoratively, need not be a time consuming task (13), but it will need to be repeated for later pregnancies, as women tend to lapse into their former dietary habits after delivery.

It must not be forgotten that there are almost certainly a number of environmental factors that trigger off NTD. Folic acid may be an important factor in the British Isles, other factors may be relatively more important elsewhere. The search for further triggers must continue.

Summary

Three studies are reported based on women resident in Glamorgan and Gwent who had had a child with a neural tube defect (NTD).

In the first study the contemporaneous inter-pregnancy diet of 415 was recorded and compared to the history of their diet during the pregnancy which had resulted in a fetus with a NTD. A blood sample was taken and analysed for folates and vitamin B_{12}. The quality of these interpregnancy diets was classified into good, fair or poor, according to whether they were deficient in specific nutrients. This classification correlated with the serum and red cell folate concentrations. The quality of their diets during the relevant pregnancy had been even worse than the interpregnancy diet. A non random half of the women were advised to improve their diet before and during the next pregnancy.

Of these women 174 reported 186 pregnancies in time for a further diet study and blood samples before the 11th week of pregnancy. Of the women counselled to improve their diet 80% had done so, compared to 10% of those not counselled. There were eight recurrences of NTD in 186 pregnancies, all these eight mothers were still receiving a poor diet during the first 2 months of pregnancy.

In the second study the interpregnancy diets of 244 women who had had a child with a NTD were compared to the diets of their own sisters and a group of professional women. The diet of the index cases was worse than that of either control group. There were 176 pregnancies in these women with five NTDs. All these five mothers had poor diets during the first 2 months of the pregnancy resulting in a NTD.

In the third study, the women who had taken part in the first study were allocated at random to preconceptional treatment using either 4 mg folic acid daily or a placebo. There were 123 women who returned pregnant claiming to have taken the tablets, 60 on folate, 63 on placebo. Of those allocated to folate 16 were considered to be non-compliers. There were six recurrent NTDs: four amongst the placebo group, two amongst the non-compliers and none amongst the treated group.

It is concluded that folic acid supplementation may be effective in preventing recurrences. It is recommended that a further trial is required to examine whether folic acid supplementation can be efficiently administered to other groups of women before conception and if so whether it would be effective in preventing neural tube defects. At the same time, improvement in the maternal diet by dietary education in school and dietary counselling for women at increased risk of neural tube defect should not be neglected.

References

1. Beck, F. (1981). Personal communication.
2. Bradshaw, J., Weale, J. and Weatherall, J. (1980). Congenital malformation of the central nervous system. *Population Trends* **19**, 13–18.

3. Burke, B. S. (1947). The dietary history as a tool in research. *J. Am. Dietet. Assoc.* **23**, 1041–1046.
4. Carter, C. O. (1974). Clues to the aetiology of neural tube malformations. *Dev. Med. Child Neurol.* **16**, Supplement 34, 3–15.
5. Chalmers, T. C. and Sacks, H. (1982). Vitamin supplements to prevent neural tube defects. *Lancet* **i**, 748.
6. Edwards, J. H. (1982). Vitamin supplementation and neural tube defects. *Lancet* **i**, 275–276.
7a. Elwood, J. H. (1980). Possible prevention of neural tube defects by periconceptional vitamin supplementation. *Lancet* **i**, 648.
7b. Elwood, J. M. and Elwood, J. H. (1980). "Epidemiology of Anencephaly and Spina Bifida", p. 23. Oxford University Press, Oxford.
8. Hibbard, E. D. and Smithells, R. W. (1965). Folic acid metabolism and human embryopathy. *Lancet* **i**, 1254.
9. Hoffbrand, A. V., Newcombe, B. F. A. and Mollin, D. L. (1966). Method of assay of red cell folate activity and the value of the assay as a test for folate deficiency. *J. Clin. Path.* **19**, 171–81.
10. James, N., Laurence, K. M. and Miller, M. (1980). Diet as a factor in the aetiology of neural tube malformations. *Zeitschrift für Kinderchirugie* **31**, 302–7.
11. Jongbloet, P. H. (1981). Neural tube defects. *Lancet* **ii**, 1291.
12. Laurence, K. M. (1983). Spina bifida and anencephaly in South Wales. *In* "Genetic and Population Studies in Wales". (P. S. Harper and E. Sunderland, eds). University of Wales Press, Cardiff (in press).
13. Laurence, K. M. (1982). Neural tube defects: a two-pronged approach to primary prevention. *Pediatrics* **70**, 648–650.
14. Laurence, K. M. and Campbell, H. (1981). Trial of folate treatment to prevent recurrence of neural tube defect. *Br. Med. J.* **282**, 2131.
15. Laurence, K. M., Carter, C. O. and David, P. A. (1968). The major central nervous system malformations in South Wales. II. Pregnancy factors, seasonal variations and social class effects. *Br. J. Prev. Soc. Med.* **22**, 212–222.
16. Laurence, K. M., James, N. and Campbell, H. (1982). Blood folate levels and quality of the maternal diet. *Br. Med. J.* **285**, 216.
17. Laurence, K. M., James, N., Miller, M. and Campbell, H. (1980). Increased risk of recurrence of neural tube defects to mothers on poor diets and the possible benefits of dietary counselling. *Br. Med. J.* **281**, 1542–1544.
18. Laurence, K. M., James, N., Miller, M., Tennant, G. P. and Campbell, H. (1981). Double-blind randomised controlled trial of folate treatment before conception to prevent recurrences of neural tube defects. *Br. Med. J.* **282**, 1509–1511.
19. MacMahon, B. and Yen, S. (1971). Unrecognised epidemic of anencephaly and spina bifida. *Lancet* **ii**, 260–261.
20. Nevin, N. C. (1980). Recurrence risk of neural tube defects. *Lancet* **i**, 1301–1302.
21. Nevin, N. C. (1981). Neural tube defects. *Lancet* **ii**, 1290–1291
22. New, D. A. T. (1978). Whole Embryo Culture and the study of Mammalian Embryos during Organogenesis. *Biol. Rev.* **53**, 81–122.
23. Record, R. G. and McKeown, T. (1949). Congenital malformations of the central nervous system I – survey of 930 cases. *Br. J. Prev. Soc. Med.* **3**, 183–219.
24. Renwick, J. H. (1982). Vitamin supplementation and neural tube defects. *Lancet* **i**, 748.
25. Seller, M. J. (1982). Nutritional supplementation and prevention of neural tube

defects. *In* "Clinical Genetics: problems in diagnosis and counselling" (A. M. Willey, T. P. Carter, S. Kelly and I. H. Parker, eds). Academic Press, London and New York.
26. Shepard, T. H., Tanimura, T. and Robkin, M. A. (1970). Energy Metabolism in Early Mammalian Embryos. *Dev. Biol.* Suppl. **4**, 42–58.
27. Smithells, R. W., Ankers, C., Carver, M. E., Lennon, D., Schorah, C. J. and Sheppard, S. (1977). Maternal nutrition in early pregnancy. *Br. J. Nutr.* **38**, 497–506.
28. Smithells, R. W., Sheppard, S. and Schorah, C. J. (1976). Nutritional deficiencies and neural tube defects. *Arch. Dis. Child.* **51**, 944–50.
29. Smithells, R. W., Sheppard, S., Schorah, C. J., Nevin, N. C. and Seller, M. J. (1981). Trial of folate therapy to prevent recurrences of neural tube defects. *Br. Med. J.* **282**, 1793.
30. Smithells, R. W., Sheppard, S., Schorah, C. J., Seller, M. J., Nevin, N. C., Harris, R., Read, A. P. and Fielding, D. W. (1980). Possible prevention of neural tube defects by periconceptional vitamin supplementation. *Lancet* **i**, 339–340.
31. Smithells, R. W., Sheppard, S., Schorah, C. J., Seller, M. J., Nevin,N. C., Harris, R., Read, A. P. and Fielding, D. W. (1981). Apparent prevention of neural tube defects by periconceptional vitamin supplementation. *Arch. Dis. Child.* **56**, 911–918.
32. Smithells, R. W., Sheppard, S., Schorah, C. J., Seller, M. J., Nevin, N. C., Harris, R., Read, A. P., Fielding, D. W. and Walker, S. (1981). Vitamin supplementation and neural tube defects. *Lancet* **ii**, 1424–1425.
33. Stone, D. H. (1980). Possible prevention of neural tube defects by periconceptional vitamin supplementation. *Lancet* **i**, 647.
34. Tanimura, T. and Shepard, T. H. (1970). Glucose Metabolism by Rat Embryos *in vitro. Proc. Soc. Ex. Biol. Med.* **135**, 51–54.
35. Tennant, G. B. and Withey, J. L. (1972). An assessment of work simplified procedures for the microbiological assay of serum vitamin B, and serum folate. *Med. Lab. Tech.* **29**, 171–181.
36. Thiersch, J. B. (1952). Therapeutic abortions with folic acid antagonist, 4-amino pteroylglutamic acid (4 amino PGA) administered by oral route. *Am. J. Obstet. Gynaecol.* **63**, 1298–1304.
37. Tuchmann-Duplessis, H. and Mercier-Parot, L. (1957). Sur l'action tératogène de l'acid X-methylfolique chez la souris. *Comptes rendues hebdomadaires des séances de l'Academie des Sciences* (Paris) **245**, 1963–1965.
38. Watt, D. J. (1977). Mechanism of development of spina bifida in the chick. PhD thesis, Aberdeen University.
39. Wilson, J. G. (1973). "Environment and Birth Defects." Academic Press, London and New York.

Acknowledgements

We are grateful to Action Research for the Crippled Child and to Tenovus for support.

Appendix 1. Dietary Enquiry Form.

DIET

Name:

Address

Breakfast	MEAT		COOKING				SALADS
		Roast	Boil	Stew	Fry		
	Beef (10)						Lettuce
	Lamb (3)						Tomatoes (5)
	Pork (3)						Cucumber
	Veal (5)						Beetroot (20)
	Chicken (3)						Celery (70)
	Ham (8)						Radishes (10)
Mid-morning	Bacon						Watercress (50)
	Liver (250)						Mustard and Cress
	Kidney (60)						Spring Onions
	Hearts (3)						Parsley (40)
Lunch	Beefburgers						
	Sausages						FRUIT
	Tinned Meat						Apples: (1)
							Cooking
	FISH						Eating
	White (50)						Bananas (10)
	Haddock						Oranges (5)
Tea-time	Kippers						Pears (2)
	Fish Fingers						Plums (2)
	Salmon (5)						Grapefruit (3)
	Sardines (2)						Grapes
							Peaches
Supper	VEGETABLES	Boil	Time	Water	Fry		Tangerines
	Cabbage (20)						Melon (6)
	Cauliflower						Raspberries (5)
Bed-time	Broccoli (30)						Strawberries (5)
	Sprouts (30)						Blackberries (12)
	Peas (20)						Blackcurrants (12)
	Beans:						Gooseberries
	Broad (0)						Rhubarb (3)
	Runner (0)						Dates (25)
Between meals	Mushrooms (20)						Figs (25)
	Spinach (80)						Prunes
	Asparagus (100)						
	Laver Bread						FRUIT JUICE
Sweets	Carrots (10)						
	Onions (10)						CANNED FRUIT
	Potatoes (20)						
Chocolates	Parsnips (20)						NUTS
	Swedes (5)						Peanuts (55)
	Turnips (4)						Salted
							Fresh
Alcohol	HOME GROWN						Almonds (45)
	VEGETABLES						Brazils (4)
							Walnuts (77)
Smoking	CEREALS						Hazel
	Cereals						
	White Bread (14)						DAIRY
	Brown Bread (35)						PRODUCTS
	Cakes (10)						Eggs (8)
	Biscuits (10)						Butter (0)
	Ryevita (30)						Milk (0)
	Pasta						Cheese (0)
	Rice (10)						
	Curries						

Appendix 2. Dietary Study Allocation of Subjects with Previous N.T.D.

Subjects visited on register 902

Subjects accepted for dietary study 442
Subjects already on folate 1
Subjects already pregnant 26

Subjects analysed in dietary study 415

Subjects refusing any tablet (0) 197
Subjects allocated to folate (A) 114
Subjects allocated to placebo (B) 104

Subjects allocated to treatment groups 415

Subjects on good diet 65
Subjects on fair diet 197
Subjects on poor diet 149
Subjects with inadequate history 4

Subjects to diet groups 415

FOLATE INTERVENTION TRIAL
ALLOCATION OF PREGNANCIES

Pregnancies reported 186
Pregnancies on no tablets (0) 56
Pregnancies reported too late (A) or (B) 7

Pregnancies admitted to folate trial 123

Pregnancies in folate group >10 μg/l (A) 44
Pregnancies in folate group <10 μg/l (A) (NC) 16
Pregnancies in placebo group (B) 63

Pregnancies analysed in trial 123

Appendix 3. All Pregnancies with Recurrence of Neural Tube Defect in Intervention Trial.

Patient No.	Diet in this pregnancy	Treatment allocation	Previous obstetric history	Year	Outcome	Reason for exclusion
86	P	NC	miss, N, An, N, miss, miss,	1973	SBC	–
154	P	NC	SBC survivor, miss	1971	An	–
149	P	B	An, SBC survivor	1973	SBC	–
265	P	B	An, N.	1974	SBC + Exomph	–
288	P	B	miss, miss, An.	1973	An	–
293(i)	P	B	An.	1974	An	–
			IN DIETARY STUDY ONLY			
99	P	O	SBC, N, N	1971	An	–
108(ii)	P	O	SBC, miss, An	1973	An	Incomplete blood chemistry
			EXCLUDED FROM BOTH DIETARY STUDY AND TRIAL			
13	P	O	An, N(masc)	1973	An + Exomph	>3/12 pregnant
91(ii)	P	B	N, SBC, miss	1973	SBC) N) twins	>3/12 pregnant
108(i)	P	O	SBC, miss	1970	An	>3/12 pregnant
214(ii)	P	A (NC)	miss, miss, miss, SBC, N(A)	1973	SBC	>3/12 pregnant
167	P	B	An, N(G), N(G)	1977	SBC	Beyond study period
201(ii)	P	A	N, An, N(A)	1977	An	Beyond study period
293(ii)	P	B	An, An	1976	An	Beyond study period

P = Poor Diet. G = Good Diet. A = Folic acid suppl. B = Placebo. O = No supplementation. NC = Folic acid non-complier. An = Anencephaly. Exomph = Exomphalos. SBC = Spina bifida cystica. miss = misscarriage. masc = mascerated. N = normal outcome.

Note: Subjects 201 and 214 had normal children when taking folate tablets under supervision, but when they became pregnant beyond the supervised period they reverted to an unsupplemented and poor diet and both fetuses had neural tube defects. Subject 167 had two normal pregnancies in the study period when she was on a good supervised diet and treated with the placebo tablet. Outside the study period she reverted to a poor diet and the fetus had a neural tube defect.

Commentary

Dick Smithells:

First Dietary Study Diets were assessed from the mothers' recollection of what they had eaten between pregnancies and in the first trimester of previous pregnancies. The recall interval ranged from a minimum of 9 months to a maximum of some years. Furthermore, the mothers obviously knew which of their pregnancies had resulted in NTD births. I cannot accept the validity of these dietary assessments.

Second Dietary Study These mothers were asked about their eating habits before marriage and during all pregnancies. This must have demanded a remarkable capacity to recall. Modification of "poor diet" to include those unbalanced by excess CHO is introduced but no evidence is adduced to suggest that these diets were deficient in folic acid or other vitamins. This is crucial to the subsequent analysis. Although all five NTD recurrences were to women on "poor" diets, only two were on poor diets as defined in the first dietary study.

Folic Acid Supplementation Study Laurence's choice of folic acid alone for supplementation may prove to have been right, but his reasons for believing that it was much more likely that the main cause (of NTD) in the British Isles was a lack of folate are not strong. They indicate that folate is likely to be important: they provide no evidence that other vitamins are not.

Women with serum folates below 10 μg/l were classified as non-compliers. No evidence is offered in support of this assumption, and studies by ourselves and others suggest that it is unlikely to be true. (My own serum folate before supplementation was 2 μg/l: after 1 week of Pregnavite forte F 1 tablet t.d.s., 4 μg/l: after 28 days supplement, 8 μg/l.) This assumption is crucial to the interpretation of results. It is difficult to accept that 27% of a group of highly motivated women failed to comply, unless the tablets made them feel unwell (not unknown with high doses of folic acid).

Replies from Nansi James:

Design Problems The validity of the dietary history rests on understanding what is aimed at in taking that history. Exact recall is impossible, but an individual's nutritional status depends on present and past food habits. It is therefore the details of the usual food *pattern* and variations that is of value. The average diet over a period (which may be considerable) is much simpler to assess where, as in these women, the individual diet varies little from week to week, season, or even year. The usual pattern at each mealtime was found to depend on the mother's way of living, e.g. no regular meal time except at 4.30 p.m. Nibbles during every other waking hour (rating poor, i.e. in *all* essential nutrients, not only in folic acid). This pattern would have been invariable since the woman gave up work (she might have had a canteen dinner at work, 5/week, previously) to bring up her family. In this area few women went out to work during this period. Food *habits* dominated the quality and balance of the diet. The check list served to clarify the usual intake. Burke claims that "the final result gives a surprisingly representative picture of the individual's average intake for any given period".

I am aware that "fair but unbalanced" is difficult to define. Such diets were not good in the intake of several essential nutrients, and in at least one other might be rated "poor". In addition we decided on arbitrary amounts of refined carbohydrate and fat before labelling the diet excess of either or both, e.g. refined carbohydrate + + + = at least 1 lb sweets and 5 bars chocolate per week and cakes, pop, icecream; fat + + + = at least daily chips plus four packets of crisps. (If we rated the *combined* fat refined carbohydrate per week as excessive, then we meant that our *total* fat and refined carbohydrate added up to at least three plus).

As Burke (1) says "The application of a detailed dietary history method shows that in pregnant women a correlation exists between dietary ratings and various objective measures of nutritional status". She studied 216 cases over 12 years and found that "the majority of infants with marked congenital malformation were born to mothers whose diets were "very inadequate". No one knows the individual's requirements for maintaining her in good health, because individual intakes vary so much that we are unable to judge the norm. But we are not concerned with the mother's needs, but what the fetus requires in order to develop normally. Any claim about the requirements of the human infant is likely to rest mainly on animal experiments, though there are a few studies (e.g. Burke) on the relation between maternal antenatal diets and the outcome of pregnancy, though the majority are based on information from antenatal clinics and therefore do not cover the first trimester.

We did not base our project pregnancy diets on their recommended values for *pregnant* women because of the belief that a mother does not need to eat more than usual early in pregnancy. Girond (3) states:

A correct equilibrium between various nutriments is important at all stages. A poor protein diet results in poor tissue differentiation. Malformations of all kinds, but most often in the CNS, results from an unbalanced diet. The lack of an essential amino acid (and of some vitamins) can lead to malformation. Experiments have shown that there must be a correct balance of nutrients, deficiency or excess of any nutrient being noxious. Deficient feeding (of animal proteins) long before gestation can affect the fetus adversely.

In *"Individual Dietary Surveys"* Marr (4) states "there is no generally accepted method of measuring the dietary intake of any free and living individual". It is important to define the objective. A detailed history of dietary *habits* furnishes important information, and, properly taken, a dietary history is of greater value than is usually appreciated. Pampiglione (5) says that in animals "fetal malformations result from a lack of balance in foods, which must provide the proper sequence of amino acid in order to build up the enzyme systems. The proportion of refined carbohydrate and fat can affect the amino acid requirements and can inhibit their absorption". A diet containing a high proportion of sweets, chocolates, cakes and soft drinks, is lacking in the proportion of vitamins and essential trace elements. Excessive proportions of lipids can be teratogenic in animals.

The only up-to-date information I have about dietary recommendations in the 1980s comes from this year's publication by the British Diabetic Association's Medical Advisory Committee (2) which states "scientific investigation has contributed less than it should to dietary theory and practice!" They recommend that *appropriate forms* of carbohydrate should make up half or more of the total energy content (i.e. calories), and that fat should be reduced to 35% – they add that this means chips not more than once a week. By the above they refer to the need for carbohydrates to be in the form of *polysaccharides* (we have called this *unrefined* carbohydrate). They mean wholemeal bread and cereals, potatoes and peas and beans (pulses). They recommend foods rich in fibre, by which they mean the above foods plus green vegetables, salads and fruit. *Refined* starches (e.g. cornflour, cornflakes) should be used sparingly, while rapidly absorbed *Mono-* and *Di*-saccharides (what we call refined carbohydrate) such as sweets, chocolates and soft drinks are best excluded from the diet.

Because of an increasing number of studies of the diets of various ethnic groups, the up-to-date idea of an "adequate" diet is no longer limited to rigid proportions of each nutrient. The fact that women seem to thrive on the crops they are able to cultivate in Third World countries is not compatible with fetal malformation rates, which are not available in some of these countries.

In recommending an optimum diet for pregnant women it is essential to focus on the needs of the fetus, and for that purpose I know of no recent recommendations that have superceded the old-fashioned ones. Criticisms should be ignored if they are based solely on the requirements for the health of the mother.

1. Burke, B. S., Feal, V., Kirkwood, S. B. and Stuart, H. C. (1943). Nutrition studies during pregnancy. *Am. J. Obstet. Gynaecol.* **46**, 38–51.

2. Final version of the dietetic recommendations for diabetics for the 1980s of the Nutrition subcommittee of British Diabetic Association's Medical Advisory Committee.
3. Girond, A. (1973). Nutritional requirements of the embryo. *World Rev. Nutrit. Diabet.* **18**, 195–262.
4. Marr, J. W. (1971). Individual dietary surveys: purposes and methods *World Rev. Nutrit. Dietet.* **13**, 105–164.
5. Pampiglione, G. (1973) Effect of metasolic disorders on brain activity. *J. Roy. Coll. Phys.* **7**, 347–364.

Chris Schorer:

The Decreasing Incidence of NTD One of the most important clues to the aetiology of NTD must lie with the cause for the decrease in prevalence of the condition in the UK and in the USA (see p. 155). Identification of any environmental change associated with this falling incidence could be important to our understanding of the aetiology of the condition. Laurence suggests that changes in dietary intake, particularly of fresh fruit and vegetables, may have contributed to the falling incidence. Unfortunately, there is no evidence to indicate that there has been an improvement in the general standard of nutrition in the UK during the last 20 years (2). The quantities of vegetables and fruit purchased, have fallen slightly during this period, although the quality eaten may have increased due to the increase in the use of frozen vegetables. Hence, with the exception of the years of poor potato crops (1975–6) when vitamin C intake fell to the lowest level for many years, intake of this vitamin has remained constant. No values are available for consumption of folic acid, but quantities of liver and green vegetables bought (both major sources of folic acid), have changed very little during the last 20–30 years. Regional, socioeconomic and seasonal differences in fruit and vegetable purchases have also persisted. Whilst reports of the National Food Survey Committee (4) of food purchased is a crude assessment of intake, especially in high risk groups, we have no other evidence that intake has changed, and so we must look elsewhere for possible explanations for the decrease in prevalence of NTD in the UK (2). The fall in incidence reported in the USA in the last 50 years (9) is over such a time scale that nutritional improvement may have contributed to the decrease.

Jongbloet (1) has raised the possibility that a decreased birth rate in the lower social class groups and in mothers who are at the extremes of the age range for bearing children, (high risk groups for NTD) could account for some of the decrease in numbers of NTD occurring in the last 10 years. However, prevalence of anencephaly has fallen in the age range 20 to 34 years (see p. 155). Another possible explanation for the change is the increase in the number of therapeutic abortions for NTD which has resulted from the increase in α-fetoprotein screening. However, this theory does not stand close scrutiny. The decrease in NTD in the population has been far in excess of any contribution that could have been made from therapeutic abortions (Chapters 5 and 6).

Folic acid and causation of neural tube defects The evidence for the suggestion made by Laurence that folic acid deficiency is the main factor in the causation of NTD in the British Isles is gaining strength. Two apparently successful intervention studies have used either folic acid alone or folic acid with other micro-nutrients. Folic acid is required for the synthesis of the bases needed for the replication of genetic information during cell division (10). Hence, cell division and neural tube closure could be compromised by folic acid deficiency.

However, not all the evidence points to a close association of folate deficiency with NTD. I am aware of no animal studies that have shown an increased incidence of NTD induced by dietary restrictions of folic acid alone; folic acid antagonists or antibiotics have been required (3). Both the increased folic acid requirement at the time of neural tube closure and lower blood folic acid levels at the beginning of pregnancies which end in infants with NTD could be mimiced by increased requirements and low levels of other micronutrients in addition to folic acid (7). There is also evidence to suggest that folic depletion may not be the main environmental factor associated with an increased incidence of NTD. Women who have very low levels of folic acid in late pregnancy and who therefore almost certainly have low levels at the time of closure of the neural tube do not show a marked increase in the incidence of the condition (4). In other words, folic acid deficiency itself seems unable to induce the condition. It requires other factors, which could be either a genetic predisposition, or a lack of other dietary components.

Certainly in biochemical terms one can implicate other vitamins. In Fig. 3 the direct involvement of a number of vitamins in the metabolism of folic acid is illustrated. Five vitamins or their metabolites are required in these processes and marginal deficiencies of several vitamins, a not uncommon feature in those taking an inadequate diet, may be as detrimental as a severe depletion of a single vitamin. The methyl-folate trap hypothesis postulated by Scott (6) would ensure a reduction in the levels of folate available for DNA synthesis even in the presence of adequate dietary supplies of folic acid if there was a deficiency of B_{12}. Low B_{12} levels would guarantee the channelling of folate into the methyl folate form which would then be excreted, rather than being returned to free tetrahydro-folate. Vitamin B_{12} has also been implicated in the aetiology of NTD (5).

Overall evidence suggests that lack of appropriate folic acid concentrations is the most likely micronutrient deficiency to affect closure of the

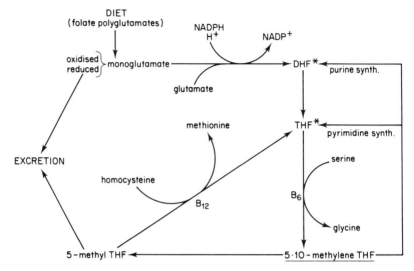

Fig. 3. The vitamins and vitamin metabolites involved in methyl group transfer in man. *Ascorbic acid is believed to help maintain folic acid metabolites DHF (dihydrofolic acid) THF (tetrahydrofolic acid) in the reduced form.

neural tube. We must however, be careful not to fall, like folic acid, into a trap, by ignoring the possible role of other vitamins such as B_{12}.

1. Jongbloet, P. H. (1981). Declining incidence of neural tube defects. *Lancet* ii, 1291.
2. National Food Survey Committee, Annual Reports (1955–79). Household food consumption and expenditure. Ministry of Agriculture Fisheries and Food. H.M. Stationary Office London.
3. Nelson, M. M. (1960). Teratogenic effects of P.G.A. deficiency in the rat. *In* "Congenital Malformations" p. 134. (G. E. W. Wolstenholme and C. M. O'Connel, eds). Ciba Foundation Symposium, Churchill, London.
4. Pritchard, J. A., Scott, D. E., Whalley, P. J. and Haling, R. F. P. (1970). Infants of mothers with megaloblastic anaemia due to folate deficiency. *J. Am. Med. Ass.* **211**, 1982.
5. Schorah, C. J., Smithells, R. W. and Scott, J. (1980). Vitamin B_{12} and anencephaly. *Lancet* i, 880.
6. Scott, J. M. and Weir, J. M. (1981). The methyl folate trap. *Lancet* ii, 337.
7. Smithells, R. W., Sheppard, S. and Schorah, C. J. (1976). Vitamin deficiencies and neural tube defects. *Arch. Dis. Child.* **51**, 944.
8. Smithells, R. W., Sheppard, S., Schorah, C. J., Seller, M. J., Nevin, N. C., Harris, R., Read, A. P., Fielding, D. W. and Walker, S. (1981). Vitamin supplementation and neural tube defects. *Lancet* ii, 1424.
9. Stein, S. C., Feldman, J. G., Friedlander, M. and Klein, R. J. (1982). Is myelomenigoale a disappearing disease. *Pediatrics* **69**, 511.

10. White, A., Handler, P., Smith, E. L., Hill, R. L. and Lehman, I. R. (1978). "Principles of Biochemistry", 6th ed. p. 1351. McGraw-Hill, London.

Replies from Nansi James: Dr Schorah says that the intake of liver and green vegetables has changed very little in the last 30 years.

He can only be referring to the Ministry of Agriculture and Fisheries reports on regional family expenditure on various foods. This is not the same as knowing what individual women eat. I found that the wife often eats much less well than the rest of the family, either because, e.g. they can only afford to buy steak for the man, or because she has a "sweeter tooth" than he has, or because she is the compulsive nibbler in the family.

Up to 1974 at any rate (I ceased trying to keep up with the literature when the Tenovus project got under way, as it would not have been possible to introduce any changes after that) ours is by far the biggest investigation of the individual diets of largely working-class mothers in any area.

Ian Leck: Although these authors have already published reports on several aspects of their study of the relationship of maternal diet to blood folate levels and pregnancy outcome in South Wales, this paper breaks new ground not only by including unpublished data on a further dietary study but also, perhaps more significantly, by clarifying that the so-called "first dietary study" and the "folate acid supplementation trial" were in fact different dimensions of a single intervention study in which each full participant was *both* (a) either given or not given dietary counselling, depending on where she lived, *and* (b) randomly allocated either folate or placebo supplementation.

This study has of course been criticized for not assessing diet more rigorously (1). However, even to have demonstrated an association between an imperfect measure of dietary sufficiency and the risk of malformation is an important achievement, or would be if the grading of diet in each women were done in a way that did not allow it to be biased by the outcome of pregnancy. Unfortunately, bias of this kind could have played a part in bringing about the finding that all eight recurrences in this study occurred in women whose first-trimester diets were graded "poor". The possibility that this grading was biased arises because although the dietary data were collected during pregnancy (when the outcome was unknown), and although the initial grading on the basis of these data was done by a worker who also did not know the outcome, one of the authors who had this information (NEJ) later reviewed the data in order to regrade as "poor" those in the "fair" grade whose diet was considered to have been unbalanced by excessive amounts of refined carbohydrates and fats. It would be incautious to

K. M. Laurence et al.

accept the reported association between recurrence and diet at its face value without hard evidence that this regrading of "unbalanced" diets neither arose out of any finding that some of the recurrences had occurred in women with this type of diet, nor was influenced in any instance by the reviewer's knowledge of the outcome of pregnancy. One would like to know how many pregnancies with recurrences and how many with a normal outcome were regraded.

. Bender, A. E. (1981). Diet and fetal neural tube defects. *Brit. Med. J.* **282**, 310.

Norman Nevin:

Evidence for Folic Acid. Several authors (Laurence *et al*; Leck and Smithells) have referred to folic acid antagonists which, when used as abortifacients induced neural tube defects in the fetus. These drugs induce striking cranial anomalies such as absent or defective ossification, misshapen bones, sutural synostosis, underdeveloped supraorbital ridges, micrognathia and severe growth retardation. However, of 12 reported cases in the literature (1–11), only two resulted in infants with a true NTD (meningomyelocoele and anencephaly) (1, 2).

. Thiersch, J. B. (1952). Therapeutic abortions with a folic acid antagonist, 4-aminopteroylglutamic acid, administered by an oral route. *Am. J. Obstet. Gynaecol.* **63**, 1298.
2. Thiersch, J. B. (1956). The control of reproduction in rats with the acid of antimetabolites and early experiences with antimetabolites as abortifacient agents in man. *Acta Endocrinol.* (Suppl.) **28**, 37.
3. Meltzer, H. J. (1956). Congenital anomalies due to attempted abortion with 4-aminopteroylglutamic acid. *JAMA* **161**, 1253.
4. Warkany, J., Beaudry, P. H. and Hornstein, S. (1959). Attempted abortion with aminopterin (4-aminopteroylglutamic acid) *Am. J. Dis. Child.* **97**, 274.
5. Emerson, D. J. (1962). Congenital malformation due to attempted abortion with aminoopterin. *Am. J. Obstet. Gynecol.* **84**, 356.
6. Shaw, E. B. and Steinbach, H. L. (1968). Aminopterin-induced fetal malformation. *Am. J. Dis. Child.* **115**, 477–482.
7. Milunsky, A., Fraef, J. W. and Gaynor, M. F. (1968). Methotrexate-induced congenital malformations *J. Pediatr.* **72**, 790.
8. Howard, N. J. and Rudd, N. L. (1977). The natural history of aminopterin-induced embryopathy. *Birth Defects Original Article Series* Volume XIII, 85–93.
9. Shaw, E. B. (1972). Fetal damage due to maternal aminopterin ingestion. *Am. J. Dis. Child.* **124**, 93–94.
10. Powell, H. R. and Ekert, H. (1971). Methotrexate-induced congenital malformations. *Med. J. Aust.* **2**, 1076–1077.

11. Brander, M. and Nusste, D. (1969). Fetopathie du a l'aminopterine avec stenose congenitale de l'espace medullaire des os tubulaires longs. *Ann. Radiol.* (Paris) **12**, 703–710.

Paedar Kirke:

Folic Acid Supplementation Study In the belief that the most valid evidence on efficacy of therapies is that derived from properly designed, executed and analysed randomized control trials, I would like to consider the trial conducted by Laurence and his colleagues (5) in some depth. This study which was conducted in South Wales is the only randomized control trial of vitamin supplementation in the prevention of neural tube defect (NTD). The important question is whether or not this trial established the efficacy of folate supplementation in reducing the risk of recurrence of NTD.

Beginning in 1969 the investigators visited 905 Welsh women who had previously had an infant with a NTD and 443 of these were considering having a further pregnancy. The women were invited to take part in a clinical trial in which they were randomized to receive either 2 mg of folate or a placebo twice daily before and during early pregnancy. Of the women entered into the trial, 123 achieved a subsequent pregnancy and were eligible "for entry to the folate analysis group"; 60 of these had been randomized to receive folate and 63 placebo.

The number of mothers entered into the trial was not specified in the earlier drafts of the paper and there was no information on withdrawals or dropouts. The results of a randomized trial should always be reported without exclusions (7) and this has been done in the final draft.

There were two NTD births in the folate group and four in the placebo group; this difference between the groups was not statistically significant. Compliance with therapy was measured in the folate group but not in those on placebo. Sixteen of the 60 mothers on folate were classified as non-compliant and both of the recurrences in the folate group were to non-compliant mothers. There were no recurrences among the 44 folate mothers adjudged to be compliant. The investigators combined the 16 non-compliers in the folate group with the placebo group and calculated that the difference in the recurrence rate between the folate compliers and the remainder (16 folate non-compliers plus 63 placebo mothers) was statistically significant ($P = 0.04$).

There is a fundamental methodological problem in the manner in which the non-compliant pregnancies were handled in the analysis of the results of this trial. If they are included with the folate group as originally randomized in an "intention-to-treat" analysis (9) the trial is negative. If they are included with the placebo group, as the authors have done, the trial is positive. So the key question is whether or not the latter approach is scientifically sound.

To combine the folate non-compliers with the placebo group is to assume that the compliers and non-compliers have the same risk status (in this case of having a recurrence of NTD) and that any difference between them in outcome can be attributed to folate alone. By the same reasoning, one would expect compliers and non-compliers of the placebo group to have identical outcomes in this (or any other) trial. We know from an important North American study (3) that this is not the case. In a large randomized clinical trial of several lipid-influencing drugs in the treatment of coronary heart disease (3), it was found that for patients on placebo therapy the mortality rate among non-compliers was 57% higher than the rate for compliers (Table 9). Furthermore, the results in Table 9 have already been corrected for 40 baseline characteristics in these patients so that the different mortality experience of the compliant and non-compliant groups cannot be explained by socio-demographic or clinical differences between them (3). Apparently, compliant patients have a considerably lower risk than non-compliant patients quite apart from any effects of treatment. As Sackett pointed out in an editorial that accompanied this publication: "Because highly compliant patients, whether they are receiving active therapy or placebo, appear destined for rosy prognoses, a comparison with their less compliant cohorts becomes a test for bias, not efficacy (8).

If Laurence and his colleagues (5) had measured compliance in the placebo group one could then compare outcomes between the folate compliers and the placebo compliers and between the folate non-compliers and the placebo non-compliers; however, larger numbers would be necessary for such an analysis to be meaningful.

Thus, combining the folate non-compliers with the placebo group is not scientifically valid and as the only unbiased analysis is by randomized assign-

Table 9. Five-year Mortality in Patients on Placebo by Compliance in the Coronary Drug Project.

	No. of patients	Death rate[a] %
Compliant	1813	16·4
Non-compliant	882	25·8

[a]Adjusted for 40 baseline characteristics. Significance of difference: $P < 0.00001$.

ment, one can conclude that this trial did not establish the efficacy of folate in the prevention of NTD. Indeed, in discussing their findings, Laurence *et al.* stated: "The use of folate as an effective prophylactic regimen to prevent NTD . . . should be further tested in a large controlled trial . . ." (5).

In a control trial investigating the efficacy of a treatment it is essential to measure compliance. If the results of a trial show no difference between a test treatment and placebo, we need to ask if the apparent ineffectiveness of the treatment is real or due to poor compliance. The investigators used the serum folate concentration to assess compliance in taking the folate tablets. They assumed that if the serum folate taken at the sixth to the ninth week of gestation was higher than 10 µg/l the woman's account of taking the tablets in the earlier part of the pregnancy could be accepted as valid. The figure of 10 µg/l as a cut-off point seems to have been chosen on a somewhat arbitrary basis. Furthermore we do not know if serum folate is a good measure of long-term compliance in taking folate tablets. The findings reported by Smithells in his paper to this Workshop (p. 60) suggest that the red blood cell folate level may be more suitable than the serum folate concentration for monitoring long-term compliance. The relationship between the pattern of folate tablet ingestion and serum and red blood cell folate levels is not clear as yet and it is hoped to investigate this in the randomized trial currently underway in Dublin. Compliance in the Dublin trial is being measured in two ways: firstly, blood vitamin levels taken at around 6 weeks' gestation (when the patient is still on the vitamin tablets) are compared with baseline values taken at randomization before the tablets are administered; secondly, each randomized mother is visited every 2 months by a research assistant who delivers a new set of tablets, takes the old box of tablets, tries to assess in a non-threatening manner whether the mother is taking the tablets and, after the visit, counts the number of tablets remaining in the old container.

Dietary studies. The dietary studies of Laurence and his colleagues are most interesting although, to this reader at least, somewhat difficult to interpret. I am impressed by the great effort which was made by Professor Laurence's team to collect dietary data on a large number of mothers on several occasions. The main finding of these studies is the association between poor maternal diet and NTD.

In his account of the first dietary study, Laurence states that all eight of the NTD recurrences occurred in those women whose diet during the first trimester was considered to be poor compared with the absence of any recurrences in the 141 mothers taking a good or fair diet. This is impressive but I should like to know for each of the eight cases whether or not the first trimester dietary assessment and its subsequent categorization into good/ fair/poor was made *before* (a) amniocentesis for α-fetoprotein measurement was carried out and (b) the outcome of the pregnancy was known either as a result of (a) or at birth? If the outcome of the pregnancy (or the likely outcome in the case of an elevated α-fetoprotein at amniocentesis) was known to the mother or the fieldworker before the dietary assessment was conducted or before the final categorization of the diet was made, one would have less confidence in the findings reported because of the well known biasing effect such knowledge would have on the assessment.

Comparing for individual mothers the diet during the first trimester of the pregnancy that ended in a NTD birth with diets during their normal pregnancies is subject to the same type of bias: the fact that she had a baby with a NTD may alter a mother's recollection of the events that preceded the birth. Furthermore, how valid are dietary assessments based on women's recollections of events which took place a number of years previously?

The method used by Laurence and his co-workers to categorize the diet has been severely criticized by an expert in nutrition (2). However, recent findings by Laurence's group (6) show a marked association between the dietary rating which they used and red blood cell folate levels. Despite the shortcomings of the method used, it appears that their dietary rating closely reflects intakes of folate-rich foods.

Finally, I would like to hear the views of the other participants on the suggestion by Barford and Pheasant (1) that a dose of 4 mg of folate (as used in the Welsh trial) "would have some inhibitory effect on dihydrofolate reductase" and that this might damage the fetus.

1. Barford, P. A. and Pheasant, A. E. (1981). Trial of folate treatment to prevent recurrence of neural tube defects. *Br. Med. J.* **282**, 1793.
2. Bender, A. E. (1981). Diet and neural tube defects. *Br. Med. J.* **282**, 310.
3. Coronary Drug Project Research Group. (1980). Influence of adherence to treatment and response of cholesterol on mortality in the Coronary Drug Project. *N. Engl. J. Med.* **303**, 1038–41.
4. Laurence, K. M., James, N., Miller, M., Campbell, H. (1980). Increased risk of recurrence of pregnancies complicated by fetal neural tube defects in mothers receiving poor diets, and possible benefit of dietary counselling. *Br. Med. J.* **281**, 1592–4.
5. Laurence, K. M., James, N., Miller, M. H., Tennant, G. B. and Campbell, H. (1981). Double-blind randomized controlled trial of folate treatment before conception to prevent recurrence of neural-tube defects. *Br. Med. J.* **282**, 1509–11.
6. Laurence, K. M., James, N. and Campbell, H. (1982). Quality of diet and blood folate concentrations. *Br. Med. J.* **285**, 216.
7. Peto, R. (1978). Clinical trial methodology. *Biomedicine* **28** (special issue), 24–36.
8. Sackett, D. L. (1980). The competing objectives of randomized trials. *N. Eng. J. Med.* **303**, 1059–60.
9. Sackett, D. L. and Gent, M. (1979). Controversy in counting and attributing events in clinical trials. *N. Engl. J. Med.* **301**, 1410–2.

Don Naismith: The relationship between social class, the quality of the diet and the incidence of NTD is very plausible. In this paper, however, as in most clinical studies in which nutritional status is regarded as an important factor, the assessment of food intake was qualitative rather than quantitative. It is not possible, therefore, to relate nutrient intake to Recommended Intakes, and to decide whether dietary deficiencies were likely to have existed in any of the subjects. The evaluation of the diets was based on somewhat outdated concepts about what constitutes a "good" or a "poor" diet, with much emphasis on the source of protein (animal or vegetable) and on the nature of the dietary carbohydrate ("refined" or "unrefined"). Since there is no evidence that NTD arises from the interaction of deficiencies of a large number of different nutrients (including amino acids and minerals) or that dietary fibre is in any way involved, this method of diet classification is largely irrelevant. It should be noted, for example, that a diet with a high proportion of carbohydrate (starch) has not only been blessed by the Royal College of Physicians (1976), but is surely desirable for a pregnant woman whose fetus relies almost exclusively on glucose for its energy supply, and the much-maligned potato provides a major part of the ascorbic acid in the average British diet. This vitamin is reported to be low in the leucocytes of mothers whose fetuses have NTD.

The promising results of the folic acid supplementation experiment make this form of diet classification even less useful, at least for the investigation of NTD. Animal protein (all meats), milk and milk products, and most fruits, major components of the "good" diet, contain very little folic acid (3–7 μg/100 g), whereas beans (30–100 μg) and white bread (35 μg) are rather good sources. What really matters is the level of consumption of foods rich in folate and, as pointed out by Laurence, the method of cooking. It was not entirely serendipidous that the system of classification worked. The "good" diets, composed of a great variety of foods, provided a generous intake of folic acid, whereas the "poor" diets, lacking in green vegetables and fruits, provided very little.

The education of mothers-to-be is clearly an important path to be explored in the prevention of NTD and appropriate diet counselling or diet supplementation of mothers at risk may be the most effective procedures at this time. When evidence for the role of vitamins in the prevention of NTD has been consolidated, however, a less orthodox approach might be considered. I believe the epidemic of overweight infants in the early 1970s disappeared largely as the result of countless articles published in the popular press and in women's magazines. Spina bifida may then be ready for the mass media.

1. Royal College of Physicians/British Cardiac Society (1976). Prevention of coronary heart disease. *J. Roy. Coll. Phys.* **10**, 213.

Reply from Nansi James: We never claimed that potatoes were harmful, only that a diet consisting largely of chips contained too much fat to be regarded as well balanced.

There was also a large number of descriptions of the affected pregnancy being the worst one as regard appetite, nausea and vomiting, and malaise. Why should one not believe such statements, especially when the sibling control, when asked about the Index's eating habits, verified these statements? Those who had a craving for sweet things during the affected pregnancy were equally corroborated by their sibs.

John Edwards: This paper is central to the issue, since Laurence and his colleagues, more than anyone, has pursued this condition against the disciplined background of an extensive experience, followed by various studies directed to the population, the family, and the general environment, including the dietary environment. This work started in the 1960s.

In spite of the encumbrance of obscure models, redundant neologisms, and archaic statistical procedures, he has pursued the thread of hope through these semantic jungles and both promoted this malformation to the status of a deficiency disease, provisionally defined the specific nutrient, and tested this possibility.

Laurence's paper, like many voyages of discovery, can be criticized in detail, but the central thread seems to lead through the maze. It is tortuous, but I do not think it is disconnected.

Some of its vagaries are due to the difficulties of the terrain, and some due to the inappropriate words and statistical procedures which have been advanced and recommended by those less experienced with working with raw data.

Laurence's paper first introduces his claim that there is a causal thread, and that it can be exploited to reduce the incidence of this disorder. He then suggests that there is a need for a controlled trial, of the general form of the planned MRC trial.

This is a serious *non-sequitur*, for environmental modifications based on knowledge should not be judged exclusively by statistical procedures which are based on ignorance.

In order to vindicate a claim of successful environmental modification which is not self-evident, some measure of response is needed. In self-evident procedures, as using water for dehydration, or blood for haemorrhage, it is usual to act without explicit validation. In the case of folic acid supplementation, and the claim of a major response, Laurence should not be criticized for the inevitable difficulties of working with a basically healthy population with limited resources and, initially, uncertain aims.

The correspondence following the uncontrolled trials has made public some criticisms, but the crucial criticism – the detailed specification of a population within which predisposition to neural tube defect and one aspect of maternal behaviour would be sufficient to deceive experienced investigators claiming a major effect – remains unmade. The evaluation of what we may term the "epidemiological landscape" is not a formal statistical problem, as Sir Ronald Fisher so sadly demonstrated in his contemptuous dismissal, on sound statistical grounds, of the work of Doll and Hill relating lung cancer to smoking. The landscape may be irregular, foggy, or even crevassed. However, we have no reason to expect mirages to be sufficiently seductive to justify the expense of independent surveyors.

There are fields of medicine in which experts do not agree on what is best, as in leukaemia therapy, or how some apparent therapy can act, as in aspirin and coronary heart disease, or isoniazid and psychosis. In such fields the well-worn machinery of the therapeutic trial, with its null hypotheses and significance tests, may in the short term advance knowledge faster than causal inquiry.

In essence, the decks are cleared of the medley of fact and fiction to allow the calculus of ignorance to make a clean sweep. Large numbers are needed, and errors, which are cummulative on serial trials, will arise at a defined rate for falsely accepting useless remedies, and at an undefined rate for rejecting useful remedies. In spite of logical inconsistencies the system seems to have worked well both in advancing therapy and prevention and in protecting patients from useless treatments.

However, where there is a substantial body of knowledge this "clearing of the decks" is not acceptable since it requires what is known to be discovered again. Where outcome is known, and diagnosis objective and obvious, placing the whole test population on a regime rather than half, will double the numbers, increase the precision of any estimate fourfold, and greatly increase the information per unit cost due to administrative simplicity. It will be a trial but not a controlled trial. Efficiency will be achieved at the cost of bias. However, a little bias is hardly a problem beyond the resources of simple arithmetic and common sense when large effects are claimed in a common disorder. The efficiency of this approach does not seem to have been appreciated. Basically, n patients can be divided into two groups of $n/2$ and the variance of their differences will be proportional to $n/4$. Laurence, like Smithells, used one group, and a comparison with historical and collateral data. A controlled trial would have had an efficiency of 25%, or needed four times as much data to reach the same precision of estimation. These estimates may have been biased but could hardly have been sufficient to explain so marked effect.

There are four major decisions to be made:

(1) Should women who have had an affected child be supplemented.
(2) Is pre-conceptional supplementation necessary.
(3) Should all potentially fertile women be supplemented.
(4) Should the whole population be supplemented.

The weight of evidence would suggest "yes" for the first, observational studies exploiting sudden or unexpected conceptions for the second, and causal studies for the third and fourth. None are amenable to randomized trials.

This is part of the wider problem of whether epidemiology can exist as a subject divorced from subject matter, in the same way as accountancy can cover any financial activity in any currency, or whether it can only flourish if rooted in a solid background of clinical or laboratory experience, as in the similar case of grammar and language. There are areas of medicine in which ignorance is sufficiently deep to justify ignoring the distractions of a little knowledge, and this is a field in which various Medical Research Council trials have made a major contribution. Unfortunately, there is no satisfactory "calculus of knowledge", and the weighing of complex evidence cannot be entirely numerical. Common sense cannot be quantified.

Felix Beck: In spite of the experimental findings of Cockroft (1979), it was decided for a variety of reasons to choose folic acid as the most likely candidate in dietary deficiency to produce neural tube defects. A folic acid supplementation study was embarked upon and this showed, as before, that folate considerably reduced (perhaps even eliminated) recurrence of neural tube defects. However, over a quarter of the women allocated to take folate failed to comply with the tablet regime and, as an epidemiological trial, the findings are no more than suggestive because the probability of such a distribution occurring by chance using the single-tail t test was equal to $0·04$.

The author argues that, due to poor compliance in his own studies and criticism which can be launched against the choice of controls in the Pregnavite forte F supplementation trial, the time has not yet come for supplementation of the population on a large scale at least before the results are confirmed by a well controlled study.

I would agree with this conclusion and suggest that the methodology now available for growing rat embryos throughout the period of neural tube formation in human serum (within their extra-embryonic membranes) provides an excellent opportunity for a direct biological assay of the blood from women at risk. Measurement of morphological and biochemical parameters of rats growing in such human sera is now highly sophisticated and it should be possible to detect not only frank malformations but also growth retardations and changes in DNA/RNA ratios. Results could be quickly obtained and would form a rational basis for proceeding to clinical trials from a point of greater information than is available to us at the moment.

Laurence also draws attention to the possibility of other environmental factors causing neural tube defects. These are well known and the very magnitude of success obtained in the preliminary trials give pause for thought. In addition, though I do not know of any detailed papers on the subject, dietary levels in certain countries where neural tube defects are prevalent must be lacking in vitamins to a far greater degree than that occurring in this country.

Folic acid is an important compound *particularly* in the early stages of embryonic growth. DNA synthesis is impossible without it and the *rate* of growth of the early embryo is higher by a factor of thousands than later in fetal or postnatal life.

Therefore folic acid is certainly a good vitamin to test initially.

One could hardly conceive of it being unimportant though it may be synthesized by the extra-embryonic membranes. The Krebs cycle enzymes are less important for reasons already given. It may be as mentioned earlier that the extraembryonic membranes may synthesize certain of these compounds (or store them).

1. Cockroft, D. L. (1979). Nutrient requirements of rat embryos undergoing organo-genesis *in vitro. J. Reprod. Fertil.* **57**, 505–510.

Norman Nevin: Despite the severe criticism of the manner in which Laurence assessed the diet of the participants in the studies, he makes a major contribution in demonstrating an association between "poor diet" and NTDs.

It would be important for the Workshop also to resolve the question of the teratogenicity of vitamin A. To my knowledge, there is no evidence that vitamin A in the dose found in Pregnavite forte F is teratogenic in either man or any animal. Several mothers in the Northern Ireland study have been on Pregnavite forte F for as long as 1½ to 2 years without any adverse affects.

It is also difficult to understand in women who would presumably be highly motivated that such a high proportion failed to follow the recommended treatment regime.

Mary Seller: Is it not fair to criticize the relevance of animal findings to man, by saying that in the past there has been evidence from epidemiological and/or clinical studies of other possible specific environmental factors which might be of aetiological importance but which subsequently have been found not to be so. The vitamins/maternal nutrition/folic acid are just another in this succession, but as further studies are being undertaken look now as if they are worth pursuing even further.

What exactly is the direct evidence that closure of the neural tube is dependent on oxygen gradient, which in turn is dependent on sufficient folate? This is of vital importance. (It should perhaps be mentioned that there is experimental evidence in animals that orderly closure of the neural tube is critically dependent on many factors.)

Please discuss the validity of serum folate levels with a cut-off of 10 μg/l for testing compliance – especially since a placebo patient who had an NTD child had a folate level of 10 μg/l. Low folate levels in the "so-called" non-compliers could be explained by poor absorption of folate and this could be the "key" to why this group had the recurrence of NTD. All the patients had been asked if they had taken their tablets and they had all said "yes". Is it justified to disbelieve so many?

I think it is an overstatement to say that the folate supplementation study *demonstrates* that folate unavailability to the embryo. I do not believe it demonstrates this.

I think it should be mentioned that what the study does demonstrate is the importance of a good diet in preventing NTD.

Nicholas Wald: I refer to Tables 2 and 3 of Laurence's paper. One hundred and eighty six pregnancies were studied, 109 in one area, 77 in another. The first area received dietary counselling and three pregnancies resulted in a neural tube defect (3/109), in the second area no special counselling was given and five pregnancies resulted in a neural-tube defect (5/77). Although the study was too small to be sure that the results did not arise by chance they do suggest an effect of counselling. It would be helpful to know whether the counselled area was selected at random, and perhaps see some actual data on the frequency of NTD risk factors in the two areas.

It would be of interest to have some details of how the diets were classified into the various groups.

My comments on the folic acid supplementation study are given above.

Could the comments on the changing "incidence of NTD" be supported by evidence? It would be helpful to distinguish between estimates of incidence and birth prevalence.

Hubert Campbell: It seems to me that there are two types of future intervention trials being discussed; (a) a trial of aetiology to test whether

NTD is the result of a folate deficiency in a specific group of high risk mothers who have had a previous malformation and whether this can be remedied by successful folate therapy; and (b) a trial of preventive measures whether the administration of any form of preventive treatment which has to be started before conception and continued into pregnancy for 3 months would ever be effective in the population groups at high risk or even at low risk of NTD.

Within either of these proposed trials there would be a serious problem of the ethics of a control form of treatment. My own feeling is that an inert control substance would no longer be justified. I am even doubtful whether Pregnavite forte (without folate) could be justified, but I can accept that many may be able to justify such a regimen.

We must not lose the point that Laurence *et al.* did not find any NTD defects in women who had an adequate diet as judged by Dr James' standards.

Even if a population intervention trial proved ineffective the real issue seems to be health education. How can we ensure that girls and young women take an adequate diet from adolescence onwards? Would it be advisable to consider an additive in some common food, as has been done with iodine in salt, fluorine in water, the B vitamins in bread and vitamin C in margarine. The women on inadequate diets are going to be precisely the same women who fail to respond to health education and will not take a preconceptional pill.

Editor's note: *See also comments on Laurence's paper in Appendix III.*

Prevention of Neural Tube Defects in an Area of High Incidence

NORMAN C. NEVIN

Department of Medical Genetics,
Queen's University of Belfast

Neural tube defects (NTDs), anencephaly and/or spina bifida, are amongst the commonest and the most tragic of congenital malformations in man. Despite extensive research over the past few decades, the precise cause(s) still remains unknown. With such a common birth defect, it would be easy to become discouraged of ever being able to prevent its occurrence, or at least, to reduce its prevalence. However, some recent research suggests that dietary counselling and periconceptional vitamin supplementation in women at risk of an infant with an NTD, may prevent recurrence. This paper describes some of the research which has been undertaken in Northern Ireland, an area with a high prevalence rate of NTDs.

Prevalence of Neural Tube Defects

A high prevalence rate of NTDs has been reported for Northern Ireland (16, 17, 40, 60). The study of Stevenson *et al.* (60), was based on hospital births only, raising some doubt as to whether the high prevalence rate was real or partly due to preselection of such cases for management in specialist obstetric hospitals. However, the investigations of Elwood and Nevin (16, 17) and Nevin *et al.* (40), which were based on the total population at risk and

128 *Norman C. Nevin*

employed multiple sources of ascertainment, probably reflected the true prevalence rate of NTDs.

In Belfast, for the period 1964 to 1968, the 41 351 total births were followed until each resulted in death (stillborn or infant death), or survival at age when ascertained (1–5 years). Of this quinquennial cohort, 151 (41 males and 110 females) had anencephalus, 185 (76 males and 109 females) had spina bifida, and 24 (5 males and 19 females) had anencephalus and spina bifida (Table 1). The prevalence rate of anencephalus, which included infants with anencephalus and spina bifida was 4·2 and of spina bifida 4·5 per 1000 total births (16), giving an overall prevalence rate of NTDs of 8·7 per 1000 total births.

Similarly, for Northern Ireland, there was a high prevalence rate of NTDs (40). In the period 1974 to 1976, a total of 686 infants was identified with NTDs among 79 783 total births. Of this cohort, 245 had anencephalus alone or associated with spina bifida, 319 had spina bifida, 71 had isolated hydrocephalus, and 51 had other NTDs such as iniencephaly. The prevalence rate of anencephalus was 3·1, and of spina bifida 4·0 per 1000 total births (Table 1), giving an overall prevalence rate of 7·1 per 1000 total births.

Table 1. Prevalence Rate of Neural Tube Defects.

	Belfast 1964–8	Northern Ireland 1974–6
Births (live and still)	41 351	79 783
Anencephalus alone or with spina bifida	175 (4·2)	245 (3·1)
Spina bifida	185 (4·5)	319 (4·0)
Anencephalus and spina bifida	360 (8·7)	564 (7·1)

Figures in brackets = prevalence per 1000 total births.

From 1964 to 1980, the overall prevalence rate of anencephalus was 3·1 and of spina bifida 3·4 per 1000 total births. In Northern Ireland, as in Liverpool (44) and in England and Wales as a whole (2), there has been a substantial decline in the prevalence rate of NTDs in the last decade (41). A highly significant decrease was observed in the prevalence rate of anencephalus. In 1964, the prevalence rate was 3·6, and in 1980, the figure was 1·7 per 1000 total pregnancies (Table 2). For spina bifida, the decrease in prevalence rate was not as striking. In 1964 and in 1980, the prevalence per 1000 total births was 4·0 and 2·0 respectively. Owens *et al.* (44) also observed that the decline was greater for anencephaly than for spina bifida.

Table 2. Prevalence of Anencephaly and Spina Bifida per 1000
Total Births Northern Ireland, 1964–1980.

Year	Total live and stillbirths	Prevalence per 1000 total births Anencephaly	Spina bifida
1964	35 025	3·6	4·0
1965	34 550	3·8	3·9
1966	33 778	3·4	3·3
1967	34 009	3·7	3·4
1968	33 714	3·3	3·4
1969	32 930	3·0	3·4
1970	32 551	3·3	3·2
1971	32 227	3·4	3·6
1972	30 428	3·2	3·6
1973	29 589	2·5	2·8
1974	27 534	2·8	4·2
1975	26 505	3·0	4·5
1976	26 639	2·5	3·2
1977	25 747	2·5	3·7
1978	26 482	1·7	3·1
1979	28 426	1·8	3·0
1980	28 581	1·7	2·0
Total	518 715	3·1	3·4

Prenatal diagnosis and selective abortion of affected pregnancies is an obvious explanation for the decline in prevalence rate of NTDs at birth. However, the decline in prevalence rate began in 1971 (Fig. 1) before screening for NTDs by serum alphafetoprotein was available. In Northern Ireland, although mothers who have had an infant with an NTD have access to prenatal diagnosis, routine serum alphafetoprotein screening of antenatal patients is not available. In 1973 to 1980, 507 births with anencephalus were registered, and 32 pregnances terminated because of an anencephalic fetus. If these pregnancies had continued to term, the prevalence rate at birth would have been 2·46 instead of the observed rate of 2·31 per 1000 total births. Prenatal diagnosis with selective abortion, therefore, only influenced the prevalence rate by the order of 6·1%. In the same period, 725 spina bifida infants were born, and there were 17 fetuses with spina bifida from 15 pregnancies which had been terminated. If these pregnancies had continued to term, the prevalence rate at birth would have been 3·37 instead of the observed rate of 3·30 per 1000 total births. Prenatal diagnosis with selective abortion, therefore, only influenced the prevalence rate by the order of 2·1%. Clearly, prenatal diagnosis and selective abortion is not a major factor in the decline in prevalence of NTDs, although it does play some part.

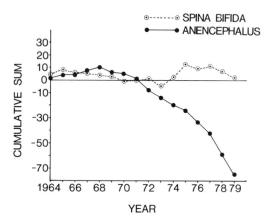

Fig. 1. Cumulative sum for spina bifida and anencephalus in Northern Ireland, 1964–79.

The cause(s) of the decline in prevalence rate of NTDs are unknown. Over the years the prevalence rate of NTDs has shown peaks and troughs (15). In North America, there was a marked rise in prevalence rate in the 1930s followed by a gradual decline. There is some evidence that a similar phenomenon occurred in the British Isles over the same period. At present prevalence rates in the British Isles may reflect another nationwide decline. It is important that attention should be given to the current secular trend in prevalence rates before attributing the decline in prevalence rate to intervention programmes.

Aetiology of Neural Tube Defects

The aetiology of NTDs, as with other common malformations, appears to be multifactorial with an important genetic factor and a substantial environmental component. Carter (4) states that family studies of NTDs indicate that their occurrence depends on the additive effects of several minor abnormal genes (i.e. polygenic inheritance) and environmental factors that also may be multiple. An accumulation of these aberrant genetic and environmental factors can be tolerated by the fetus to a point (the "threshold"), beyond which there is a risk of a malformation. Carter (5) concludes that "little is yet known about the mechanisms by which the genetic predisposition acts, or of the environmental factors involved".

The multifactorial inheritance model has a number of very specific predictions (see p. 155). Recently, some inconsistencies between the model predictions and the observed data have been noted (35). The reason may be that there is likely to be aetiologic heterogeneity for NTDs including single gene loci and chromosomal abnormalities (23). The paper by Toriello, Warren and Lindstrom (63) suggests strongly that some NTDs occur as an X-linked mutation. Possible autosomal dominant inheritance has been also suggested for some NTDs (22). However, at present, most NTDs probably have a multifactorial threshold determination.

Over the past 12 years, several studies in Northern Ireland have been undertaken to identify the possible genetic and the environmental components involved in the aetiology of NTDs. These investigations have suggested several possible environmental factors.

Geographic Variation

The prevalence rate of NTDs in communities in the United Kingdom and Ireland is shown in Table 3. The prevalence rate shows a marked geographical gradient, which steadily increases from the south and east to the north and west; for example, in Northern Ireland the prevalence rate of NTDs is double that for the whole of England and Wales. This geographic gradient has been confirmed by several reliable studies (12, 19, 50, 61). Even within Northern Ireland, the geographical gradient persists, with a prevalence rate of spina bifida of 4·8 per 1000 total births in the western area compared with 3·8 per 1000 total births in the eastern area which includes Belfast.

This geographic variation may depend on a variety of factors. Biosocial factors such as maternal age and parity could be important. In England and

Table 3. Prevalence Rate of Neural Tube Defects.

Centre	Year of study	Reference	Year of publication	Rate per 1000 total births
Birmingham	1950–2	McKeown and Record	1960	4·8
Liverpool	1960–4	Smithells	1968	6·5
Southampton	1958–62	Williamson	1965	5·1
Leicester	1953–62	Moss	1964	4·9
Glasgow	1964–5	Wilson	1970	5·6
Dublin	1963–4	Coffey	1973	8·3
Cork	1962–6	Spellman	1970	4·2
Belfast	1964–8	Elwood and Nevin	1973	8·7
Northern Ireland	1974–6	Nevin *et al.*	1978	7·7
South Wales	1956–62	Carter *et al.*	1968	7·6
England and Wales	1964–72	Rogers and Weatherall	1976	3·5

Wales, family size is smaller and the prevalence rate of NTDs lower. However, differences in regional parity and maternal age between birth populations at risk accounted for less than 5% of the excess of the anencephalus rate in Northern Ireland over that of England and Wales (14). In South Wales, from an analysis of the geographic variation of neural tube malformations, Richards, Roberts and Lloyd (47) also concluded that biosocial factors such as parity did not explain the marked geographical differences.

It has been suggested that the geographic variation of NTDs may be related to the quantitative differences in local water supply. Fedrick (19) collected data on anencephalus and on water supply from ten different areas in the United Kingdom. She found that the frequency of anencephalus was negatively correlated with the total hardness, calcium content, and pH of the local waters. There was a tendency for the prevalence rate of anencephalus to decrease as the hardness of water increases. However, in South Wales, softer water was associated with the poorer rather than the more prosperous areas, so that the correlation may be secondary and reflect more the socioeconomic status of the population (33). These authors concluded that the "water" factor may be a pointer to some as yet unidentified specific teratogen in the non-specific poverty complex. Detailed investigations of other individual regions in the United Kingdom did not confirm the association of NTDs with water supply (21).

There is much evidence to indicate a high proportion of embryos with NTDs are aborted spontaneously. Roberts and Lowe (49) have estimated that the total spontaneous abortion rate may be as high as 78%. Nishimura (43) has demonstrated that as many as 90% of all NTDs are lost early in pregnancy. In an investigation of the regional variation in the prevalence rates of NTDs, Roberts and Lloyd (48) found an inverse relation between previous spontaneous abortion rates and prevalence rate. They suggested that there is probably little or no difference in the incidence of NTDs shortly after conception and that the observed differences at birth are due to a greater prenatal mortality rate among malformed embryos in areas with a low prevalence rate. An attempt was made to examine this hypothesis by comparing the rate of spontaneously aborted fetus in Northern Ireland, an area with a high prevalence rate (34), with that in South-East England, an area with a low prevalence rate (10). In the latter, 3·6% of complete conceptuses which miscarried had an NTD, whereas the corresponding figure in Northern Ireland was 4·9%. Table 4 shows the outcome of pregnancies in embryos with an NTD alive at 8 weeks gestation after the last menstrual period.* In Northern Ireland, some 51·1% of affected embryos were miscarried (8–27 weeks) compared with 62·5% in South-East England. The difference in the percentage of affected fetuses in the communities is

Table 4. Outcome of Pregnancy in Embryos with Neural Tube Defects alive at eight weeks after last Menstrual Period.

	Estimated % of affected embryos with indicated outcome of pregnancy	
	Northern Ireland	South-East England
Abortions (8–27 weeks)	41·5 (51·1)	53·5 (62·5)
Stillborn (after 27 weeks)	38·6 (24·1)	22·3 (18·7)
Liveborn	19·9 (24·8)	24·2 (18·7)

Figures originally given in ref (34) are listed first, followed in brackets by figures recalculated by I. Leck (see footnote).

small and unlikely to account for the marked difference in the prevalence rate at birth. The striking geographic variation in prevalence rates of NTDs in the United Kingdom still awaits a satisfactory explanation.

Socio-economic Effect

In the United Kingdom, a consistent epidemiological feature of NTDs has been the association with social class; women of lower socioeconomic status have the greatest risk of having children with NTDs (12, 16, 19, 64, 66). The prevalence rate of NTDs has been as much as two to four times higher in social classes IV and V births, compared with women of social class I and II. A similar observation has been made in several other countries (18, 20, 24, 37, 38). The association of prevalence rate of NTDs with social class persists, even when other factors such as maternal age, parity, and geographic region, are controlled (19). In the Belfast study (16), a definite association was observed between social class and prevalence rate of all NTDs. Consid-

---

* Leck has re-examined the data of MacHenry *et al.* (34). There was an overestimation of the number of affected births per 1000 conceptuses in Northern Ireland. In computing the numbers affected, live and stillborn infants were analysed as two separate groups, as if they had been expelled during different parts of pregnancy, which introduced an error because the stillbirth rate at the time of Stevenson's survey (2·6%) was not the same as the rate that applied to the Northern Ireland series in Table 4 (1·3%). This error is overcome by estimating the number of affected live and stillbirths per 1000 conceptuses that would have occurred if the latter stillbirth rate had applied in Stevenson's series. Among the miscarried cases of NTDs in the series from South-East England, two-fifths of those that were karyotyped had chromosomal anomalies and were excluded from the data on which the percentages in Table 4 were based. In Northern Ireland, as cytogenetic studies were not available, all cases were included. This discrepancy has been corrected, where the figures given for the south-east England include cases with chromosomal anomalies. These corrections result in an increase in the estimate of miscarriage rates for both series and a reduction in the stillbirth rate among NTDs in Northern Ireland.

eration of anencephalus and spina bifida separately showed that the social class effect for spina bifida was similar to that of anencephalus (Table 5).

The association of prevalence rate of NTDs with socioeconomic status may be secondary to other environmental factors such as housing condition and maternal nutrition. In Belfast, some of these factors have been examined. The prevalence rate of NTD in the poorer areas of the City was higher than in "better-off" areas. For example, in "inner" Belfast with the oldest housing, the prevalence rate of NTDs was 11·8 compared with the overall prevalence rate of 8·7 per 1000 total births. Indeed, in some areas of "inner" Belfast with marked social and environmental deprivation, the prevalence rate was as high as 19·1 per 1000 total births (17). In addition, it was also possible to examine the association of the prevalence rate of NTD with overcrowding using an index based on the number of persons per room. The prevalence rate rises as the degree of overcrowding increases (17). In a family with an overcrowding index of two or more the prevalence rate was 12·9, compared with 8·5 per 1000 total births in families with an overcrowding index of one. In addition, the survival of spina bifida infants was reduced in families of lower socioeconomic status. Spina bifida infants born to mothers resident in "inner" Belfast, fared much worse than those in "outer" Belfast, with 18·9% and 39·5% respectively, being alive at one year.

Table 5. Prevalence Rate of Neural Tube Defects with Social Class.

	Prevalence rate per 1000 total births		
	Anencephalus	Spina bifida	Both defects
Social Classes I and II	2·46	2·74	5·20
Social Class III	4·87	4·67	9·54
Social Classes IV and V	3·81	4·58	8·39

Dietary Factors

Many authors, because of the higher prevalence rates in poorer communities, have suggested that dietary factors may be involved in the aetiology of NTDs (3, 27, 28, 32). Among the dietary factors suggested as causes of NTDs, in recent years potatoes have received most attention. In 1972, Renwick (46a) proposed that specific but unidentified factor(s) present in potato tubers, possibly induced by the potato blight fungus, *Phytophthora infestans*, might be the causal factor(s) and claimed that 95% of all neural tube defects could be prevented by the avoidance of potatoes during early pregnancy. Initially, some experimental support for the potato theory had been provided by Poswillo, Sopher and Mitchell (45) who found midline malformations of the cranium in four of eleven embryos of female marmosets fed with blighted potatoes. Supplementary experiments, however, failed to reproduce these defects (46).

In Northern Ireland, a trial of potato avoidance in women with at least one previous infant with anencephalus and/or spina bifida was undertaken in a direct attempt to test Renwick's (46a) hypothesis, that 95% of NTDs is preventable by the avoidance of potatoes during early pregnancy (42). Although the numbers involved in the study were small and allocation to the groups was non-random, the investigation failed to support the concept that short-term avoidance of potatoes before conception and throughout the early weeks of pregnancy in women who had had a previous NTD infant reduces the recurrence risk. In the group of women on a potato-free diet, of 23 pregnancies which went to term two infants had NTDs (8·7%); whereas in the group of women on a non-potato-free diet, of 56 pregnancies which went to term, two had NTDs (3·6%) (Table 6). This study and some case reports (30, 31) indicated that short-term potato avoidance in women with a previous NTD infant failed to prevent the recurrence of the malformation. There is no doubt that Renwick's (1972) hypothesis directed attention to the role of diet in the aetiology of NTDs.

Among the possible environmental factors involved in the aetiology of NTDs, maternal nutrition has been a main suspect. The effect on offspring of maternal nutritional deprivation has been demonstrated in the study of the Dutch famine of 1944/1945 (59). The cohort of conceptions exposed to the famine during the first trimester of pregnancy experienced a sharp increase in stillbirths, and also of first week deaths. In addition, there was an increase (not significant) of central nervous system anomalies. Among this cohort, there were eight cases of spina bifida and hydrocephalus, whereas only four cases would have been expected (62). Recently, Laurence *et al.*

Table 6. Outcome of the study Pregnancy in the Potato-free and non-Potato-free Groups.

| | Outcome of pregnancy | | |
	Spontaneous abortion	Normal liveborn	Infant with NTD
Potato-free group (n = 27)	4	22^a	2 (8·7%)
Non-potato-free group (n = 61)	5	55^a	2 (3·6%)

$P = 0·58$. [a] Included a twin pregnancy.

(29) have demonstrated a relationship between poor diet in the mother and the recurrence rate of NTDs, and suggested that dietary counselling would reduce the recurrence risk of NTD.

Attention also has been directed to specific dietary factors which may be important in the aetiology of NTDs. In a prospective study of blood vitamin levels in first trimester pregnancy, Smithells, Sheppard and Schorah (53) found that mean blood levels of serum folate, red cell folate, white blood cell vitamin C, and riboflavin values were lower in six mothers who gave birth to infants with central nervous system malformations than in controls. They considered the possibility that minor deficiencies of one or more vitamins might contribute to the causation of NTDs. This hypothesis was examined by an intervention study in women who had previously borne an infant with an NTD (54, 55, 56). This study included women from Northern Ireland. The results demonstrated that in women who received vitamin supplementation (Pregnavite forte F) for at least 28 days before conception and until the second missed menstrual period, that the recurrence of NTDs, compared with unsupplemented women, was significantly reduced. The authors concluded that the most straightforward explanation is that vitamin supplementation had prevented some NTDs in the women at risk. However, they emphasized that it cannot be regarded as proved and indicated that further studies were required.

In the publication of the details of the first group of supplemented women (55), several alternative interpretations for the beneficial effect were considered. In Northern Ireland, continuing studies of periconceptional vitamin supplementation with Pregnavite forte F of women with a previous infant with an NTD have resolved some of these alternative explanations. It was suggested that a group of women with a naturally low recurrence risk had unwittingly selected themselves for supplementation. Social class may be a specific factor related to the recurrence risk of NTDs. As NTDs have an association with social class, it was suggested that the recurrence risk may be lower in social classes I and II, than in social classes III, IV, and V (39). The recurrence risk of NTDs among sibs of patients with anencephalus and/or spina bifida in relation to social class is shown in Table 7. Thus, if more women of higher social classes had been included in the fully supplemented group and as they have a lower recurrence risk, this would accentuate the recurrence difference in the fully supplemented and unsupplemented groups.

Although there were fewer women of social class I, II, and IIIN (29%) in the unsupplemented group than in the fully supplemented group (43%), a significant difference in NTD recurrence favourable to vitamin supplementation still existed when only social classes IIIM, IV, and V, in both fully and unsupplemented groups were considered. Examination of the social class in

Table 7. Recurrence of Neural Tube Defects among Sibs of Index Patients with Anencephalus and/or Spina Bifida in relation to Social Class.

Social class	Prevalence of NTDs per 1000 total births	Recurrence risk among sibs per 1000
I and II	5·33	54·55
III	9·54	89·78
IV and V	8·39	93·37
Total	8·71	88·73

the fully supplemented and the unsupplemented groups in Northern Ireland shows no significant difference (χ^2 = 6·06, d.f. = 3, 0·20>P>0·10) (Table 8).

A further specific factor related to recurrence risk is the geographic area (7, 11). In the first cohort (54, 55), there was an excess of unsupplemented women from Northern Ireland, an area with a high prevalence rate of NTDs, and it could be argued that this may have weighted the unsupplemented group with high recurrence risk women. Examination of the data from Northern Ireland alone has shown this to be unlikely. Combination of the data relating to the two cohorts shows an apparent beneficial effect of periconceptional vitamin supplementation within Northern Ireland (Table 9). The lower recurrence rate in fully supplemented compared with unsupplemented women is significant (P<0·0367) by Fisher's exact method. Of 241 unsupplemented women, there were 12 (5·2%) infants/fetuses with an

Table 8. Comparison of Supplemented and Unsupplemented Women Social Class, Northern Ireland.

Social class	Supplemented	Unsupplemented
I and II	43 (28·5)	56 (24·3)
IIIN	26 (17·2)	25 (10·9)
IIIM	54 (35·8)	108 (47·0)
IV and V	28 (18·5)	41 (17·8)
Total	151[a]	230[b]

[a] Two husbands in HMS Forces. [b] Three husbands in HMS Forces and eight whose occupation was unknown. Figures in brackets are percentages.

Table 9. Periconceptional Vitamin Supplementation Northern Ireland.

	Total number of study pregnancies in which infant/fetus examined	Number of pregnancies with infant/fetus with NTD
Unsupplemented group (n = 241)	233[a]	12 (5·2%)
Fully supplemented group (n = 153)	139[a]	1 (0·7%)

[a] Includes five twin pregnancies; also excludes one patient with a normal amniotic fluid AFP lost to follow-up, and 12 spontaneous abortions which were not examined. [b] Fourteen spontaneous abortions not examined excluded. Figures in brackets are percentages P = 0·0367.

NTD among 233 infants and fetuses examined. There were five twin pregnancies. Thirteen pregnancies were excluded because one woman who had a normal amniotic fluid AFP was lost to follow up and 12 pregnancies ended as spontaneous abortions which were not examined. Of 153 fully supplemented women, there was one (0·7%) infant with an NTD, among 139 infants and fetuses examined. Fourteen pregnancies which resulted in spontaneous abortions were not examined; these were excluded. No claim has been made that fully supplemented and unsupplemented were equally at risk, but some evidence from the Northern Ireland studies would indicate that the supplemented mothers did not have a naturally low recurrence risk of infants with NTDs. In the potato-avoidance study (42), as Edwards (13) points out, the women who were treated with a potato-free diet had a higher recurrence risk (8·7%) of NTDs than the women on a non-potato-free diet (3·6%). Further, in the periconceptional vitamin supplementation study, women who withdrew or were excluded from the group recruited for supplementation had a recurrence risk similar to those women who were in the unsupplemented group. On September 30, 1981, when recruitment to the second cohort study stopped, a total of 293 women, had agreed to participate in the study (Table 10). Of these 293 women, 118 withdrew or were excluded from the study; 66 women had not become pregnant by the end of the study, 44 women were excluded because they had taken the vitamin supplementation erratically or had stopped taking the tablets. Five women were excluded because the previous affected infant was discovered to have a non-NTD lesion; one woman moved to another region and two women did not start taking vitamin supplementation until after the time of closure of the neural tube. On September 30, 1982 a complete follow-up of the 118 women who were excluded or who had withdrawn was achieved.

Of the 66 mothers who had not conceived, 38 subsequently became

Table 10. Number of supplemented and unsupplemented women with reasons for withdrawals and exclusions.

Recruited for supplementation	293	
Withdrawals and exclusions	118	
Supplemented		
Total	184	
Fully	153	(1/139)
Partially	31	(0/31)
Withdrawals and exclusions		
Erratic or discontinued supplementation	44	(0/16)
Moved to another region	1	(0/1)
Previous affected infant non-NTD	5	(0/3)
Failed to conceive	66	
Started tablets after closure of the neural tube	2	(1/2)
Unsupplemented	241	(12/233)

Brackets = number of NTDs/number of infants and fetuses examined.

pregnant and have been included in the supplemented group of cohorts 2 and 3. The remaining 28 mothers are still being supplemented. Of the other 50 women, 27 had not had any further pregnancies. Of the 23 who had become pregnant, the outcome was as follows – 21 normal infants, one spontaneous abortion which was not examined, and one infant with anencephalus. Thus the recurrence risk in the women who were excluded or withdrew from the supplemented group was 4·5% compared with 5·2% in the unsupplemented women.

Another explanation for the beneficial effect of vitamin supplementation was that something other than the vitamins had reduced the incidence of the NTDs in the group of mothers receiving treatment. Some recent work has demonstrated an association between an essential element deficiency in the mother and congenital malformations of the central nervous system. Hurley and Shrader (25) experimentally have shown that zinc deficiency causes NTDs in offspring of pregnant animals. In a large prospective study of 245 primigravidas, Jameson (26) found that five of the eight mothers who had infants with congenital malformations had low zinc values in early pregnancy. An association between anencephaly and low maternal plasma zinc has been reported (8). Recently, Soltan and Jenkins (57) have shown that plasma zinc concentration was significantly lower in maternal blood of 54 women giving birth to congenitally abnormal babies either within 24 h or 24 months previously.

Recently, we have determined essential elements, zinc, copper, and magnesium in amniotic fluid in the mid-trimester from three groups of pregnancies (Nevin, Sungkur and Merrett, unpublished data). The three groups were: (1) 50 pregnancies which led to normal infants; (2) 31 pregnancies in which the fetus had an NTD; and (3) 12 pregnancies in which the fetus had a chromosomal abnormality or an X-linked recessive disorder. The mean amniotic fluid zinc and copper values were significantly higher in the NTD group. There was no significant difference in the amniotic fluid magnesium values in the three groups (Table 11). The high amniotic fluid zinc and copper in the pregnancies in which the fetus had an open NTD may reflect some abnormality in the metabolism of these essential elements or may be secondary to an open NTD. We have also examined the zinc level in the hair of newborn infants with NTDs and in the scalp and pubic hair of their mothers at term. Compared with normal newborn infants the hair zinc values were lower in the infants with NTDs (Nevin, unpublished data).

Although the significance of abnormalities in essential elements in the aetiology of NTDs is far from clear, further studies in this area would be important. In addition to iron, calcium and vitamin content, Pregnavite forte F also contains 13 other ingredients (1). Although to our knowledge, Pregnavite forte F does not contain essential elements such as zinc or copper, it is possible that they may influence the absorption of essential elements.

Table 11. Mean Amniotic Fluid Zinc, Copper and Magnesium in Normal, Neural Tube Defects and other Congenital Malformations.

Group	Zinc μg/ml	Amniotic fluid Copper μg/ml	Magnesium m mol/l
Normal (n = 50)	0·088	0·117	0·601
NTDs (n = 31)	0·356	0·164	0·622
Other malformations (n = 12)	0·122	0·132	0·590

Future

Further investigations of the prevention of neural tube defects by periconceptional vitamin supplementation are needed to answer some of the unresolved problems:

(1) It remains to determine the role of individual vitamins, their dose, and the importance of the time of administration. The mothers with NTD infants have generally poor diets and are thus probably deficient in most nutrients. It would appear more appropriate to provide multivitamin preparations. However, some evidence also suggests

that a beneficial effect may be obtained with folic acid alone. It will be necessary to undertake studies to compare the efficiency of each preparation.

(2) If NTDs are preventable by vitamin supplementation why is it that in some mothers there is a failure to prevent the recurrence of an infant with an NTD? The obvious explanation is that of non-compliance by these mothers. However, it is most probable that vitamin deficiency is only one of the environmental factors in the cause of NTDs and possibly other as yet unidentified environmental factors may play a role.

(3) It is also important to identify women other than those who have had an infant with an NTD who might have an increased risk. One obvious group of women would be the sibs of women who have had an affected child. The risk of having an NTD infant in this group is approximately twice that for the general population. Such "at risk" mothers could be easily identified through genetic counselling centres. However, this would still leave the majority of pregnancies unprotected. In the long-term the answer lies in improving the overall diet of the population by health education and, perhaps, supplementing milk or water with vitamins.

References

1. Ancil, R. J. (1981). Quoted in Smithells, R. W., Sheppard, S., Schorah, C. J., Seller, M. J., Nevin, N. C., Harris, R., Read, A. P. and Fielding, D. W. Apparent prevention of Neural Tube Defects by periconceptional vitamin supplementation. *Arch. Dis. Child.* **56**, 911–918.
2. Bradshaw, J., Weale, J. and Weatherall, J. A. C. (1980). Congenital malformations of the central nervous system. *Population Trends* **19**, 13–18.
3. Carter, C. O. (1973). Diet and congenital defects. *Brit. Med. J.* **1**, 290–291.
4. Carter, C. O. (1974). Clues to the aetiology of neural tube malformations. *Dev. Med. Child Neurol.* **16**, 3–15.
5. Carter, C. O. (1976). Genetics of common single malformations. *Brit. Med. Bull.* **32**, 21–26.
6. Carter, C. O., David, P. A. and Laurence, K. M. (1968). A family study of major central nervous system malformations in South Wales. *J. Med. Genet.* **5**, 81–106.
7. Carter, C. O. and Roberts, J. A. F. (1967). The risk of recurrence after two children with central nervous system malformations. *Lancet* **i**, 306–308.
8. Cavdar, A. O., Arcasey, A., Baycu, T. and Himmetoglu, O. (1980). Zinc deficiency and anencephaly in Turkey. *Teratology* **22**, 141.
9. Coffey, V. P. (1973). Monitoring of congenital defects. *J. Irish Med. Assoc.* **66**, 127–130.
10. Creasy, M. R. and Alberman, E. D. (1976). Congenital malformations of the central nervous system in spontaneous abortions. *J. Med. Genet.* **13**, 9–16.

11. Editorial (1980). Vitamins, Neural Tube Defects and Ethics Committees. *Lancet* **ii**, 1061–1062.
12. Edwards, J. H. (1958). Congenital malformations of the central nervous system in Scotland. *Brit. J. Prev. Soc. Med.* **12**, 115–130.
13. Edwards, J. H. (1982). Vitamin supplementation and neural tube defects (letter). *Lancet* **i** 275–276.
14. Elwood, J. H. (1970). Anencephalus in the British Isles. *Dev. Med. Child Neurol.* **12**, 582–591.
15. Elwood, J. M. and Elwood, J. H. (1980). "Epidemiology of Anencephalus and Spina Bifida", p. 107. Oxford University Press, Oxford.
16. Elwood, J. H. and Nevin, N. C. (1973). Factors associated with anencephalus and spina bifida in Belfast. *Brit. J. Prev. Soc. Med.* **27**, 73–80.
17. Elwood, J. H. and Nevin, N. C. (1973). Anencephalus and spina bifida in Belfast (1964–1968). *Ulster Med. J.* **42**, 213–222.
18. Emanuel, I. and Sever, L. E. (1973). Questions concerning the possible association of potatoes and neural-tube defects and an alternative hypothesis relating to maternal growth and development. *Teratology* **8**, 325–332.
19. Fedrick, J. (1970). Anencephalus and the local water supply. *Nature* **227**, 176–177.
20. Field, B. (1978). Neural tube defects in New South Wales, Australia. *J. Med. Genet.* **15**, 329–338.
21. Fielding, D. W. and Smithells, R. W. (1971). Anencephalus and water hardness in south-west Lancashire. *Brit. J. Prev. Soc. Med.* **25**, 217–219.
22. Fineman, R. M., Jorde, L. B., Martin, R. A., Hasstedt, S. J., Wing, S. D. and Walker, M. L. (1982). Spinal dysraphia as an autosomal dominant defect in four families. *Am. J. Med. Genet.* **12**, 457–464.
23. Holmes, L. B., Driscol, S. G. and Atkin, S. L. (1976). Etiologic heterogeneity of neural tube defects. *New Eng. J. Med.* **294**, 365–369.
24. Horowitz, I. and McDonald, A. D. (1969). Anencephaly and spina bifida in the Province of Quebec. *Can. Med. Assoc. J.* **100**, 748–755.
25. Hurley, L. S. and Shrader, R. E. (1972). Congenital malformations of the nervous system in zinc-deficient rats. *Int. Rev. Neurobiol.* Supplement **1**, 7–51.
26. Jameson, S. (1976). Variations in maternal serum zinc during pregnancy and correlation to congenital malformations, dysmaturity, and abnormal parturition. *Acta Med. Scand. Suppl.* **593**, 21–37.
27. Knox, E. G. (1972). Anencephalus and dietary intakes. *Brit. J. Prev. Soc. Med.* **26**, 219–223.
28. Laurence, K. M., Carter, C. O. and David, P. A. (1968). Major central nervous system malformations in South Wales. II Pregnancy factors, seasonal variation and social class effect. *Brit. J. Prev. Soc. Med.* **22**, 212–222.
29. Laurence, K. M., James, N., Miller, M. and Campbell, H. (1980). Increased risk of recurrence of pregnancies complicated by fetal neural tube defects in mothers receiving poor diets and possible benefit of dietary counselling. *Brit. Med. J.* **281**, 1592–1594.
30. Lorber, J., Stewart, C. R. and Ward, A. M. (1973). Alpha-fetoprotein in antenatal diagnosis of anencephaly and spina bifida. *Lancet* **i**, 1187.
31. Lorber, J. (1974). The potato trial. *Link* **30**, 7. (Association for Hydrocephalus and Spina Bifida.)
32. Leck, I. and Rogers, S. C. (1967). Changes in the incidence of anencephalus. *Brit. J. Prev. Soc. Med.* **21**, 177–180.
33. Lowe, C. R., Roberts, C. J. and Lloyd, S. (1971). Malformations of the central nervous system and softness of local water supply. *Brit. Med. J.* **2**, 357–361.

34. MacHenry, J. C. R. M., Nevin, N. C. and Merrett, J. D. (1979). Comparison of central nervous system malformations in spontaneous abortions in Northern Ireland and in south-east England. *Brit. Med. J.* **1**, 1395–1397.
35. Melnick, M. (1979). Current concepts of the etiology of central nervous system malformations. *Birth Defects: Original Article Series* **XV(3)**, 19–41.
36. Moss, B. J. L. (1964). Congenital abnormalities in Leicester, 1953–1962. *Med. Officer* **112**, 79–82.
37. Naggan, L. and MacMahon, B. (1967). Ethnic differences in the prevalence of anencephaly and spina bifida in Boston, Massachusetts. *New Eng. J. M.* **277**, 1119–1123.
38. Nesbit, D. E. and Ziter, F. A. (1979). Epidemiology of myelomeningocele in Utah. *Dev. Med. Child Neurol.* **21**, 754–757.
39. Nevin, N. C., Johnston, W. P. and Merrett, J. D. (1981). Influence of social class on the risk of recurrence of anencephalus and spina bifida. *Dev. Med. Child Neurol.* **23**, 155–159.
40. Nevin, N. C., McDonald, J. R. and Walby, A. L. (1978). A comparison of Neural Tube Defects identified by two independent routine recording systems for congenital malformations in Northern Ireland. *Int. J. Epidemiol.* **7**, 319–321.
41. Nevin, N. C. (1981). Neural tube defects (letter). *Lancet* **ii**, 1290–1291.
42. Nevin, N. C. and Merrett, J. D. (1975). Potato avoidance during pregnancy in women with a previous infant with either anencephaly and/or spina bifida. *Brit. J. Prev. Soc. Med.* **29**, 111–115.
43. Nishimura, H. (1969). Incidence of malformations in abortions. *In* "Congenital Malformations" (F. C. Fraser and V. A. McKusick, eds), pp. 275–283. Excerpta Medica, Amsterdam.
44. Owens, J. R., Harris, F., McAllister, E. and West, L. (1981). 19-year incidence of neural tube defects in area under constant surveillance. *Lancet* **ii**, 1032–1035.
45. Poswillo, D. E., Sopher, D. and Mitchell, S. (1972). Experimental induction of foetal malformation with 'blighted' potato: a preliminary report. *Nature* **239**, 462–464.
46. Poswillo, D. E., Sopher, D., Mitchell, S., Coxon, D. T., Curtis, R. F. and Price, K. R. (1973). Investigations into the teratogenic potential of imperfect potatoes. *Teratology* **8**, 339–347.
46a. Renwick, J. H. (1972). Hypothesis: Anencephaly and spina bifida are usually preventable by avoidance of a specific but unidentified substance present in certain potato tubers. *Brit. J. Prev. Soc. Med.* **26**, 67–88.
47. Richards, I. D., Roberts, C. J. and Lloyd, S. (1972). Area differences in prevalence of neural tube malformations in South Wales. A study of possible demographic determinants. *Brit. J. Prev. Soc. Med.* **26**, 89–93.
48. Roberts, C. J. and Lloyd, S. (1973). Area differences in spontaneous abortion rates in South Wales and their relation to neural tube defect incidence. *Brit. Med. J.* **4**, 20–22.
49. Roberts, C. J. and Lowe, C. R. (1975). Where have all the conceptions gone? *Lancet* **i**, 498–499.
50. Rogers, S. C. (1969). Epidemiology of stillbirths from congenital abnormalities in England and Wales, 1961–1966. *Dev. Med. Child Neurol.* **11**, 617–629.
51. Rogers, S. C. and Weatherall, J. C. (1976). Anencephalus, spina bifida and congenital hydrocephalus. England and Wales 1964–1972. *In* "Studies on Medical and Population Subjects No. 32." Office of Population Censuses and Surveys, London.
52. Smithells, R. W. (1968). Incidence of congenital abnormalities in Liverpool (1960–64). *Brit. J. Prev. Soc. Med.* **22**, 36–37.

53. Smithells, R. W., Sheppard, S. and Schorah, C. J. (1976). Vitamin deficiencies and neural tube defects. *Arch. Dis. Child.* **51**, 944–950.
54. Smithells, R. W., Sheppard, S. S., Schorah, C. J., Seller, M. J., Nevin, N. C., Harris, R., Read, A. P. and Fielding, D. W. (1980). Possible prevention of neural tube defects by periconceptional vitamin supplementation. *Lancet* **i**, 339–340.
55. Smithells, R. W., Sheppard, S. S., Schorah, C. J., Seller, M. J., Nevin, N. C., Harris, R., Read, A. P. and Fielding, D. W. (1981). Apparent prevention of neural tube defects by periconceptional vitamin supplementation. *Arch. Dis. Child.* **56**, 911–918.
56. Smithells, R. W., Sheppard, S. S., Schorah, C. J., Seller, M. J., Nevin, N. C., Harris, R., Read, A. P., Fielding, D. W. and Walker, S. (1981). Vitamin supplementation and neural tube defects. *Lancet* **ii**, 1425.
57. Soltan, M. H. and Jenkins, D. M. (1982). Maternal and fetal plasma zinc concentration and fetal abnormality. *Brit. J. Obstet. Gynaecol.* **89**, 56–58.
58. Spellman, M. P. (1970). A five-year survey in Cork of spina bifida and hydrocephaly. *J. Irish Med. Assoc.* **63**, 339–342.
59. Stein, Z., Susser, M., Saenger, G. and Marolla, F. (1975). "Famine and Human Development: The Dutch Hunger Winter of 1944/1945". Oxford University Press, London.
60. Stevenson, A. C., Johnston, H. A., Stewart, M. I. P. and Golding, D. R. (1966). Congenital malformations. *Bull. World Health Org.* **34**, Supplement, pp. 1–127.
61. Stocks, P. (1970). Incidence of congenital malformations in the regions of England and Wales. *Brit. J. Prev. Soc. Med.* **24**, 67–77.
62. Susser, M. and Stein, Z. (1980). Prenatal diet and reproductive loss. *In* "Human Embryonic and Fetal Death" (I. H. Porter and E. B. Hook, eds), pp. 183–196. Academic Press, London and New York.
63. Toriello, H. V., Warren, S. T. and Lindstrom, J. A. (1980). Brief communication: Possible X-linked anencephaly and spina bifida – report of a kindred. *Am. J. Med. Genet.* **6**, 119–121.
64. Williamson, E. M. (1965). Incidence and family aggregation of major congenital malformations of the central nervous system. *J. Med. Genet.* **2**, 161–172.
65. Wilson, T. S. (1970). Congenital malformations of the central nervous system among Glasgow births 1964–1968. *Health Bull.* **28**, 32–38.
66. Wilson, T. S. (1971). A study of congenital malformations of the central nervous system among Glasgow births, 1964–1968. *Health Bull.* **29**, 79–87.

Commentary

Dick Smithells: As Nevin has been a member of our research group it is not surprising that I have few comments to offer.

Potatoes. I agree that experiments have not supported the potato hypothesis, although Poswillo *et al.* produced cranial vault defects in marmosets by feeding an extract of blighted potatoes to the pregnant mothers (1).

Zinc Deficiency and NTD. In my own paper I refer to the action of intestinal folate conjugases on dietary polyglutamates. It is interesting to note that these conjugases are zinc-dependent. Nevin says, "the high amniotic fluid zinc and copper . . . signifies . . . some abnormality in the metabolism of these essential elements may play a role . . .". Alternatively, are zinc and copper levels raised for the same reason that AFP is raised? Zinc plays an important part in the healing of granulation tissue.

We have offered vitamin supplements to a few women with minor degrees of spina bifida or spina bifida occulta. Numbers are so far very small but this is another high risk group.

Nevin suggests that ". . . the answer lies in improving the overall diet of the population by health education". How effective will this be, and how long will it take? Could the desired effect be achieved more quickly and on a wider scale by food additives?

1. Poswillo, D. E., Sopher, D. and Mitchell, S. (1972). *Nature* **239**, 462–464.

Ian Leck:
Abnormalities of hair zinc concentration in mothers of newborn infants with spina bifida. This is the title of a paper by Bergmann *et al.* (1). They found that:

(a) Mean hair zinc levels were higher in mothers of cases than in control mothers.
(b) During pregnancy the level rose in the mothers of cases but fell in the control mothers.
(c) The levels in mothers and offspring were directly correlated in the cases but not in the controls.

They noted that in previous work, increased hair zinc had been reported in cases of extreme zinc deficiency!

1. Bergman, K. E., Makosch, G. and Tens, K. H. (1980). *Am. J. Clin. Nutr.* **33**, 2145–2150.

Chris Schorer:
The Role of Zinc in NTD. The possible role of zinc in the aetiology of NTD (5) raises the question of the importance of the different nutrients used in any supplementation. Interrelationships of different vitamins will be considered in more detail elsewhere (comments on the paper by Laurence) but here it would be appropriate to consider the possible role of zinc.

The association between decreased maternal zinc and increased risk of NTD has been outlined (see p. 127). In biochemical terms, zinc can certainly be implicated in these defects. Thymidine kinase, DNA and RNA polymerase, enzymes required for DNA synthesis and therefore neural tube closure, require zinc as a co-factor (1). In addition, zinc is also said to be involved in the absorption of folic acid as it is required by the enzyme which converts the polyglutamate form of the vitamin to the absorbable mono-glutamate (5). However, there is also a close association between folic acid and zinc in the diet (correlation coefficient, $r = 0 \cdot 7418$; the fifth highest correlation of folate with 30 food constituents, unpublished observations). In consequence, low zinc levels may be implicated in the causation of NTD, not because of any direct effect of the trace element itself, but because of its association with a low folate concentration in the mother. Alternatively, low levels of both folate and zinc could act synergistically to encourage poor DNA metabolism and prevent neural tube closure.

The high zinc concentration in the amniotic fluid surrounding NTD-affected fetuses may, as Nevin suggests, indicate disturbed fetal metabolism of this element. However, presumably many materials are released into the amniotic fluid (e.g. alphafetoprotein) when there is an open NTD lesion. As zinc is largely intracellular and protein-bound (2), increased amniotic fluid concentrations may only reflect a release of intracellular zinc and zinc binding proteins from the neural tube lesion.

Recurrences of NTD in the Multivitamin Supplemented Group. In the intervention studies, the finding of recurrences in women believed to be fully supplemented (see p. 53) suggests that in these women the environmental factor is not corrected by the dietary treatment used because, either the genetic factor is too dominant or the environmental factor is different in these women. With regard to dietary factors, vitamin B_{12}, not present in Pregnavite forte F has been implicated in the causation of NTD (4). Alternatively, some women susceptible to NTD may have higher vitamin requirements than others because of differences in metabolism, but none have yet been identified (see p. 53). As far as the genetic predisposition is concerned it seems probable that maternal/fetal genetic and structural factors must be important in the aetiology of the condition, especially when it is remembered that low maternal folic acid levels themselves do not automatically predispose women to NTD, as shown by a failure to find an increased incidence of the condition in women with megaloblastic anaemia of pregnancy (3).

Because of the apparent complexity and individuality of the interrelationships of environmental and genetic factors in the causation of NTD, the application of the animal studies described by Seller (see p. 1) and Beck (see p. 23) become increasingly important for, as they point out, these models are far more amenable than women to metabolic and dietary manipulations.

1. Hunt, I. F., Murphy, N. J., Gomez, J. and Smith, J. C. (1979). Dietary zinc intake of low-income pregnant women of Mexican descent. *Am. J. Clin. Nutr.* **32**, 1511.
2. Kiely, M., Scott, B. and Bradwell, A. R. (1981). Zinc status and pregnancy outcome. *Lancet* **i**, 893.
3. Pritchard, J. A., Scott, D. E., Whalley, P. J. and Haling, R. C. P. (1970). Infants of mothers with megaloblastic anaemia due to folate deficiency. *J. Am. Med. Ass.* **211**, 1982.
4. Schorah, C. J., Smithells, R. W. and Scott, J. (1980). Vitamin B_{12} and anencephaly. *Lancet* **i**, 880.
5. Tamura, T., Shane, B., Baer, M. T., King, J. C., Margen, S. and Stokstad, E. L. R. (1978). Absorption of mono- and poly- glutamyl folates in zinc-depleted man. *Am. J. Clin. Nutr.* **31**, 1984.

Paedar Kirke: I enjoyed Nevin's paper and, particularly, his review of the research work on epidemiological and preventive aspects of neural tube defects (NTD) in Northern Ireland. The demonstration that the risk of recurrence of NTD varies with the incidence of the condition and with social class (1) is an important recent contribution from Nevin's team.

I agree fully with Nevin's statement that further confirmation of the apparent beneficial effect of vitamin prophylaxis is needed. But confirmation will not come merely by repeating what Nevin, Smithells and their colleagues have already been doing because of the scientific flaws in the method used (I have commented on some of these in my comments on Smithell's paper). As Meier has remarked "should the evidence at hand be subject to large potential biases, no accession of numbers or profusion of analyses will improve its relevance" (2). Randomized control trials will confirm or refute the apparent favourable effect.

I predict that there will be unanimous agreement among the participants at our meeting on one point at least – the need to improve the overall diet, not only of women at high risk of having neural tube defect births but of the childbearing population in general. Health education has an important role to play here but this objective cannot be achieved by health education alone.

1. Nevin, N. C. (1980). Recurrence risk of neural tube defects. *Lancet* **i**, 1301–2.
2. Meier, P. (1982). Vitamins to prevent neural tube defects. *Lancet* **i**, 859.

Michael Laurence: There seems to have been a fall in the incidence in Northern Ireland as in other parts of the British Isles, but this seems to have been less dramatic than the fall that has occurred in mid-Glamorgan and probably in the rest of South Wales. However, the Northern Irish figures are based on two different populations. They are for Belfast, 1964–8, and for the whole of Northern Ireland, 1974–76.

Geographical variations have been well documented. Their relationship to abortions is difficult to interpret. Probably most NTD abortions occur not after 8 weeks gestation but before. In every series so far reported the earlier the abortion material the greater the proportion of malformed fetuses with chromosome abnormalities and, more important, neural tube defects.

The direct association between neural tube defect and blighted potatoes is now not generally accepted. None the less, ingestion of large quantities of potatoes and potato products seem to be associated with high incidence of neural tube defects. This could be either because these interfere with the absorption of folic acid in diets, or displace folic acid containing foods from the diet.

Experimental zinc deficiency has long been known to precipitate neural tube defects but this has not as yet been shown to be the case in man. The finding that zinc plasma levels at the end of pregnancies are low in those ending in neural tube defects is of interest, but this should be investigated during the first trimester and not 8 months or so after the closure of the neural tube. Zinc levels in mid-trimester amniotic fluid seem to yield results which on the face of it seem to contradict the suggestion that low zinc levels might be a precipitating factor for neural tube defects. The role of zinc in the possible causation of NTD certainly warrants further study.

Future Investigations.

(1) The proposed MRC investigation will, it is hoped, confirm the beneficial effects of Pregnavite forte F or of folic acid alone, or both. If the latter is as effective as the former then there is no reason why supplementation for all pregnancies should not be adopted in the UK as folic acid is cheap and apparently completely safe in child-bearing women. Means of getting folic acid to women who do not plan their pregnancies may have to be devised.

(2) The possible role of each of the constituents of Pregnavite forte F should be investigated separately, especially that of vitamin C, enhancing the clearance of certain toxic agents, of riboflavin and pantothenic acid and the role of i-inositol.

(3) Other trigger mechanisms responsible for NTD in man (i.e. zinc deficiency etc.) should be looked for.

(4) The investigation of the pregnancies of close relatives of women who have had an NTD has already been partially carried out in south Wales (see our Second Dietary Investigation) from which more data could be made available.

Ian Leck: The epidemiology of neural tube defects have been investigated more thoroughly in Northern Ireland and South Wales than anywhere else in the area around the Irish Sea where their prevalence reaches its peak, and this paper does a useful job in reviewing the findings for Northern Ireland. There is just one matter of semantics and two or three aspects of the numerical analysis about which I have reservations.

The matter of semantics is the use of the term "incidence" – not only in this paper but also in those of Laurence and Smithells – to mean the proportion of infants born who exhibit defects. This usage, I suggest, is an example of the common fault of confusing incidence and prevalence. The *incidence* (or, more strictly, incidence rate) of any disorder is the number of people who *develop* this disorder during a given period, expressed as a proportion of those at risk of doing so. In the case of any malformation, the period in question is the period in development during which this malformation can arise; those at risk are the embryos alive during this period; and the incidence is therefore the number of embryos affected, expressed as a proportion of the total number reaching the age at which the malformation arises. The *prevalence* (or, more strictly, the point prevalence rate) of any disorder, on the other hand, is the number of people *affected* by this disorder at a point in time, expressed as a proportion of those at risk of being so. Depending on the context, the point in time may be either a particular date on the calendar or a particular point in the life cycle, e.g. birth or a particular age thereafter. Thus, the number of infants born with neural tube defects, expressed as a proportion of the total number of births, is the prevalence at birth of these defects. As these defects substantially increase the risk of miscarriage, their incidence is of course considerably higher than their *prevalence at birth* – an important reason for not confusing the two.

It is of course possible to use the data on which Nevin's Table 3 is based to estimate the extent of this difference between incidence and prevalence at birth (see Table 1 of my paper). However, there seem to be two errors in the paper (3) from which Nevin's Table 3 quotes, and these are reflected in this Table (although not, I believe in Table 1 of my chapter). These errors were as follows:

1. *Overestimation of the number of affected births per 1000 conceptuses in Northern Ireland.* For a cohort of 1000 conceptuses alive 8 weeks after the last menstrual period, the number (a) of affected conceptuses that would be expelled from the uterus during each part of pregnancy was assumed to be given by the formula $a = bc$. Here, b is the prevalence of neural tube defects per 1000 conceptuses expelled during the part of pregnancy in question and available for study; and c is the total number of conceptuses expelled during the same part of pregnancy in a Northern Ireland series of miscarriages and births assembled by Stevenson and Warnock (6), expressed as a proportion

of all the conceptuses in their series who were alive at 8 weeks' gestation. In computing the numbers affected, live and stillborn infants were analysed as two separate groups, as if they had been expelled during different parts of pregnancy, which introduced an error because the stillbirth rate at the time of Stevenson's survey (2·6%) was not the same as the rate that applied to the Northern Ireland series in Table 3 (1·3%). This error may be overcome by estimating the numbers of affected stillbirths and live births per 1000 conceptuses that would have occurred if the latter stillbirth rate had applied to Stevenson's series. Table 12 shows what the figures for Northern Ireland in Nevin's Table 3 become when this is done.

Table 12. Outcome of Pregnancy in Embryos with Neural Tube Defects alive Eight Weeks after Last Menstrual Period.

	Estimated % of affected embryos with indicated outcome of pregnancy	
	Northern Ireland	South-East England
Miscarriage (8–27 weeks)	51·1	62·5
Stillbirth (after 27 weeks)	24·1	18·7
Livebirth	24·8	18·7

2. Use of data for South East England which do not allow for cases with demonstrated chromosome anomalies. Among the miscarried cases of neural tube defects in the series from South East England, two fifths of those that were karyotyped had chromosomal anomalies and were excluded from the data on which the percentages in Table 3 are based (1). However, as nothing is said to the contrary, one assumes that all cases were included in the Northern Ireland statistics. If so, the two sets of figures in Table 3 are not comparable. This discrepancy too has been corrected in my Table 12, where the figures given for south east England include cases with chromosomal anomalies.

The main effects of these corrections are to reduce the estimated stillbirth rate among neural tube defects in Northern Ireland and to increase the estimated miscarriage rates for both series. The latter figure for Northern Ireland is increased further if it is assumed (as in my Table 1 and in all analyses of the English data) that the distribution of all pregnancies by outcome was like that given by French and Bierman (2) instead of Stevenson's.

My other reservations concern the references to the increased risk of CNS anomalies after the Dutch famine and to the high amniotic fluid zinc and copper levels reported in cases of neural tube defects. I question whether the excess of cases in children conceived at the peak of the Dutch famine was statistically significant. The relevant data (5) are shown in Table 13. The figures of eight observed and four expected cases of central nervous system anomalies after the Dutch famine do not refer to the total numbers born (which are presumably not available) but only to cases observed in males who survived long enough to be considered for National Service.

Table 13.

	Number of young men who had been born in cities affected by famine	
	Born before or conceived after famine	Conceived during four months of worst famine
CNS malformation present	48	8
CNS malformation absent	48 440	3617

χ^2 with Yates's correction $= 3 \cdot 589$. $0 \cdot 10 > P > 0 \cdot 05$.

Secondly, Nevin's evidence that amniotic fluid zinc is high in affected fetuses makes one wonder whether loss of zinc to the amniotic fluid in affected pregnancies is at least partly responsible for the low plasma zinc levels that have been observed in such cases, although this hypothesis is not supported by the report that the plasma zinc level may be low not only at the time of delivery but also two years later in the mothers of such children (4).

1. Creasy, M. R. and Alberman, E. D. (1976). Congenital malformations of the central nervous system in spontaneous abortions. *J. Med. Genet.* **13**, 9–16.
2. French, F. E. and Bierman, J. M. (1962). Probabilities of fetal mortality. *Public Health Reports (Washington)* **77**, 835–847.
3. MacHenry, J. C. R. M., Nevin, N. C. and Merrett, J. D. (1979). Comparison of central nervous system malformations in spontaneous abortions in Northern Ireland and South-East England. *Brit. Med. J.* **i**, 1395–1397.
4. Soltan, M. H. and Jenkins, D. M. (1982). Maternal and fetal plasma zinc concentration and fetal abnormality. *Brit. J. Obstet. Gynaecol.* **89**, 56–58.
5. Stein, Z., Susser, M., Saenger, G. and Marolla, F. (1975). "Famine and Human Development: the Dutch Hunger Winter of 1944–1945." Oxford University Press, New York.
6. Stevenson, A. C. and Warnock, H. A. (1958). Observations on the results of pregnancies in women resident in Belfast: I. Data relating to all pregnancies ending in 1957. *Ann. Human Genet.* **23**, 382–394.

Felix Beck: I find it difficult to understand the possibly conflicting pieces of evidence which show that Soltan and Jenkins (1982) have demonstrated that plasma zinc concentration was significantly lower in the maternal blood of women giving birth to congenitally abnormal babies whereas the mean amniotic fluid zinc and copper values were significantly *higher* in the NTD group. One is left with the thought that possibly the determination of these metals in biological fluids is somewhat inaccurate or that the two findings are unconnected and, by the same token, possibly unconnected with NTD or that the statistical tests used might have been inappropriate.

The fact that all neural tube defects are not preventable by vitamin supplementation suggests to the author that "It is most probable that vitamin deficiency is only one cause of neural tube defects and possibly other, as yet, unidentified environmental factors may play a role". I am sure this is a most important point to bear in mind and again, in this context, one would be very interested to see whether in certain groups of individuals neural tube defects are present as the sole abnormality while in others (possibly not geographically distributed in the same way) the pattern of congenital malformation differs.

Nicholas Wald: The "miscarriage hypothesis" as an explanation for the regional variation in the birth prevalence of neural tube defects is interesting. Are the data shown in Table 3 sufficient to reject the hypothesis?

It is not clear why a separate analysis of the Northern Ireland data has resolved some of the alternative explanations for the effect which could not be examined using the combined data. The observation that the beneficial effect of vitamin supplementation was present within a recruitment centre was known at the time the study was first published and could be seen from the report in the *Archives of Diseases in Childhood* (1). On p. 137 there is the statement that "when the data relating to the two cohorts are combined, the beneficial effect of periconceptual vitamin supplementation is still evident (Table 4)". Referring to "the beneficial effect" pre-judges the issue and begs the key question. There is a similar statement earlier in the paper.

It is stated at the top of p. 136 that the effect of supplementation persisted if social classes III, IV and V only are considered. This does not deal with the social class problem, since such allowance is too crude (classes III, IV and V make up most of the study population) and because social class itself is only a crude measure of the etiological factors involved. Adjusting for social class does not therefore eliminate its effects. The conclusion to be derived from the social class effect is that the results are liable to be biased by self-selection and *any* form of adjustment is likely to be inadequate.

The data relating to the concentration of essential elements in amniotic fluid are interesting, although it is necessary to bear in mind that the neural tube defect lesions may have resulted in the biochemical changes rather than the reverse.

In the discussion on future work it is suggested that continuing the current intervention study will be helpful. However, the problem with the study is not one of numbers but one of possible bias – increasing the numbers will not help. In the paper there is a presumption that vitamins are beneficial, and that we simply need to find out which vitamin is involved, the dose needed, the time of administration, etc. Since, for the reasons given in my paper, the presumption is unwarranted, the next step must logically be to investigate whether the supplementation actually works.

1. Smithells, R. W., Shepherd, S., Schorah, C. J., Seller, M. J., Nevin, N. C., Harris, R., Read, A. P. and Fielding, D. W. (1981). Apparent prevention of neural tube defects by vitamin supplementation. *Arch. Dis. Child.* **56**, 911–18.

Editor's note: For further comments on this chapter, please see Dr Schorer's comments on p. 63.

Epidemiological Clues to the Causation of Neural Tube Defects

IAN LECK

Department of Community Medicine,
University of Manchester, Manchester

As in the case of other disorders, the clues to the causation of neural tube defects yielded by epidemiological studies have been obtained by demonstrating that the frequency of these defects is related to two groups of variables. The first of these groups comprises "demographic" variables – aspects of time and space, and personal characteristics of children and their relatives, which cannot themselves be teratogenic but may serve as pointers to influences which may be. The latter influences make up the second group of variables.

For the neural tube defects, there is marked disparity between the links established with variables of these two kinds – a plethora of convincing reports of strong associations with "demographic" variables, but a dearth of good evidence incriminating specific teratogens. The main aim of this paper is to provide a brief summary of these two aspects of the literature. A full review has recently been produced by Elwood and Elwood (28).

At the outset, the senses in which certain terms are used in this paper need to be defined. "Anencephaly" includes cases in which this defect is combined with spina bifida (craniorrhachischisis), and "spina bifida" comprises all other cases of meningocoele, myelocoele and encephalocoele; many published data cannot be broken down further, and some that can suggest that craniorrhachischisis and cranial meningocoele (including encephalocoele) are epidemiologically very similar to anencephaly alone and true spina bifida, except for being much less common (82). "Prevalence" is used as shorthand for the prevalence of malformations at birth, i.e. the proportion of children born (including stillbirths) who are affected; the term "incidence" which is sometimes used in this sense should be reserved for the proportion of those at risk of a disorder who develop it, which in the case of neural tube defects means the proportion of *embryos alive at the age when these malformations arise* who are affected.

Prevalence at birth can of course be estimated much more readily than incidence, although even with the former there are problems. The most recent available British data relate to defects observed and notified by medical and nursing staff in stillbirths and infants in the first week of life. These figures show that in 1980 anencephaly and spina bifida were notified in 0·52 and 1·14/1000 total births respectively (114). However, not all cases are notified. This can most easily be demonstrated for anencephaly, the lethality of which makes the perinatal death rate virtually the same as the birth prevalence. In 1979 (the most recent year for which perinatal mortality data are available) the number of anencephalics notified was only 86% of the number in the perinatal mortality statistics (114, 123). Extrapolating from 1979 to 1980 and (less confidently) from anencephaly to spina bifida, we may estimate that in England and Wales these conditions were present in 0·6 and 1·3/1000 total births respectively in 1980.

The problem of estimating incidence has been approached in two ways. One is to measure the frequency of defects in embryos obtained when abortion has been induced shortly after the age when the defects arise, on the assumption that such embryos are representative of all those alive at this time. The other approach involves bringing together data for stillborn and other children and for miscarriages, to which must be added pregnancies terminated for fetal reasons if there are significant numbers of these (e.g. if antenatal screening for fetal defects is practised). In Table 1, British estimates based on data of the first two kinds, collected before antenatal screening became common, are compared with Japanese data for births and early induced abortions. The data are consistent in suggesting that the incidence of neural tube defects of the brain is at least three times their birth prevalence, but the contrast between the corresponding figures for spina bifida is very much less marked in the British data and more so in the Japanese. Such estimates of incidence can however only be regarded as very tentative: firstly because of difficulties in diagnosing neural tube defects in aborted embryos and fetuses (55) and secondly because those examined were not totally representative. In particular, embryos with defects severe enough to cause miscarriage within 6 weeks of conception were absent from the British series and must have been underrepresented in the Japanese one. Also, the

Table 1. Estimated incidence and prevalence of neural tube defects.

	Japanese data[a] (108, 113)	British data[b] London (9, 18)	Eastern area, Northern Ireland (95,109)
Estimated incidence/1000 embryos			
Anencephaly, exencephaly or encephalocoele	2·7 } 6·1	5·1 } 6·8	10·0 } 14·4
Spina bifida	3·4	1·7	4·4
Prevalence/1000 total births			
Anencephaly, exencephaly or encephalocoele	0·7 } 0·9	1·6 } 3·0	3·3 } 7·1
Spina bifida	0·2	1·4	3·8

[a] Incidence assumed to equal prevalence in early induced abortions. [b] Incidence assumed to equal prevalence 8 weeks after last menstrual period (calculated on the assumptions that all the embryos alive at this time were distributed by age at subsequent miscarriage or birth in the proportions reported by French and Bierman (45), and that the products of miscarriage studied were representative of all miscarriages of like gestational age).

estimates of incidence apply to a different aetiological mix of cases from that on which the prevalence statistics are based: aneuploidy, which is rare among viable cases (42), may cause two-fifths of those that miscarry (18).

Associations with "Demographic" Variables

With time, place and personal characteristics alike, neural tube defects show variations in prevalence which seem almost certain to be brought about by environmental factors – although some of these factors may be affecting not the incidence of the malformations but the miscarriage rate among the malformed.

Variations with Time

Substantial seasonal and secular trends in prevalence of neural tube defects have both been described repeatedly. Seasonal variations by factors of up to three between a peak and a trough among spring and autumn conceptions respectively have been observed in several European countries and (for anencephaly) in Canada, although they are not consistent from year to year or defect to defect. For example, trends of this kind appear to have been a feature of anencephaly but not spina bifida in Birmingham (England) during the 1940s, and in Westphalia (West Germany) during the 1950s; of both anencephaly and spina bifida over much at least of the United Kingdom during the 1950s and in England (although less consistently) subsequently; and of spina bifida but not anencephaly in Scotland, Northern Ireland and Hungary during the 1960s. Even when both defects are involved the peaks for anencephaly and spina bifida seem to differ in being centred on early and late spring conceptions respectively (19, 25, 82, 86, 90, 96, 114, 123, 129, 134, 146, 147, 154). Significant seasonal variations have not been observed in the United States, whilst in New South Wales (Australia) and Izmir (Turkey) summer conceptions may be at highest risk (4, 38, 117).

The most striking secular trends reported have been prolonged waves of high prevalence of both anencephaly and spina bifida, each with a peak higher by two thirds or more than the level before and after the wave has passed. One such wave seems to have built up during the 1920s and fallen away during the 1940s in both England and the North-eastern United States. Peaks were also witnessed in Germany in 1949, in Quebec in 1951–4, in England in 1954–5, and in Scotland and Ireland in 1960–1, but in Ontario and the North-eastern United States the trend since the 1940s has been downward (2, 23, 24, 28, 60, 67, 80, 87, 98, 129). In England and Wales the decline after 1954–5 was followed by a decade of little change, but since 1972 prevalence has again fallen, by more than half for anencephaly and somewhat less dramatically for spina bifida, the national notification rate for which has declined by two-fifths (114, 123). Antenatal diagnosis and termination of affected pregnancies seem to have accounted for only a small fraction of this decline (116).

It has been suggested that these secular variations may not have been primarily between children born in different years but between children whose mothers belonged to different birth cohorts (30). If such were the case, the years in which changes in prevalence occurred would vary substantially with maternal age, the offspring of women aged 25, for example, being affected 5 years later than those of women aged 20. Few if any of the changes that have been studied were of this kind. The wave seen in England during the 1950s seems to have affected all maternal age groups simultaneously (83), and so (with one exception) does the decline in the 1970s (Fig. 1); and although there is evidence that the changes in Scotland and the North-eastern United States that are mentioned above occurred first among the offspring of young women (1, 67, 99), the differences in timing between maternal age groups were not as great as they would have been if the same maternal birth cohort had been affected throughout. A more plausible explanation is that the changes were brought about by alterations in the environment during or shortly before the affected pregnancies, and that these alterations affected the young mothers first because such women accept innovations more quickly.

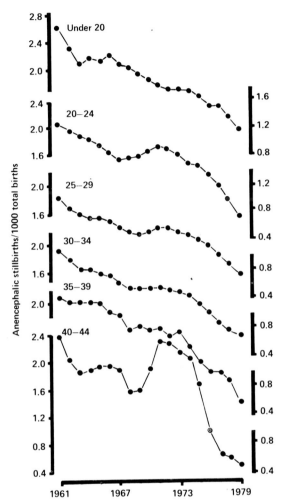

Fig. 1. Prevalence of anencephalic stillbirths (per 1000 total births) in each maternal age group, by year of birth: England and Wales 1961–79. Figures shown are single-year rates for the first and last years, and three-year sliding means for the remainder.

Variations with Place and Race

Particular caution is needed when comparing the prevalence of neural tube defects in different places, since many of the available data are based on hospital births which tend to be unrepresentative (especially where most children are born at home), and also because seasonal and secular trends like those described above are not the same everywhere and therefore alter the relationship between prevalence in different places. However, studies in hospitals and whole communities alike suggest that over the last two or three decades as a whole, the range of variation in prevalence among communities of predominantly Caucasoid origin has been of the order of threefold in the British Isles and tenfold worldwide, figures above 4/1000 births for anencephaly and the same for spina bifida having been observed in Belfast, Northern Ireland (25), and in the coal-mining valleys of South Wales (127) during the mid-1960s, whilst the figure for each defect was only about 1·5/1000 births in London at this time (9) and below 0·4/1000 in Finland (52). Apart from the British Isles, the main areas from which relatively high figures have been reported are in the eastern parts of Canada and the United States (28, 65) and in the Middle East from the eastern Mediterranean to northern India (28, 148).

It seems likely that this variability between people of Caucasoid origin in different countries is due at least partly to environmental differences. From studies of children whose forebears migrated from France to Canada (28), from various Middle Eastern countries to Israel (105), and from the regions of high prevalence in the British Isles to places of lower prevalence (9, 59, 82, 107), it seems that in the descendants of migrants, especially those of the second and later generations to be born after migration, the prevalence of neural tube defects tends to move from the levels seen in their ancestral homelands towards those found in other residents of their places of birth. The best-authenticated exceptions are perhaps the high and low rates seen in various countries in Sikhs and Ashkenazi Jews repectively (105, 107, 132, 148) – groups whose life styles may change less than others after migration.

The data available for populations of mainly non-Caucasoid descent are less extensive than for Caucasoids, but suggest that both West African Negroid and oriental Mongoloid populations living in their ancestral homelands resemble the more low-risk Caucasoid populations in their prevalence of anencephaly (around 0·5–1/1000 births) but differ from them in including fewer than half as many cases of spina bifida as of anencephaly, instead of similar numbers of each (29, 48, 82, 88, 115). In these ethnic groups too, the descendants of migrants may become more like their host communities in respect of prevalence: among black children in the United States and England (whose ancestors came mainly from west Africa), and among children of Mongoloid descent in Hawaii, the prevalence of spina bifida is within the range seen in the more low-risk Caucasoid populations, the above disparity in prevalence between defects of these two types being reduced or even reversed. However, neither defect has been observed in more than 1/1000 black children in England or the United States, even where prevalence in the white community is higher (31, 82, 103).

Variations with Personal Characteristics

The personal characteristics of children and their families that appear to be related to the prevalence of neural tube defects include the sex of the child, whether the pregnancy is single or multiple, the mother's parity and age, and the socioeconomic status and medical history of the family as a whole.

Sex ratio. In most populations that have been studied, the defects are commoner in females than in males: the ratios of prevalence in males to prevalence in females reported in large series have varied between about 0·6:1 and 0·9:1 for spina bifida, whilst the corresponding range for anencephaly is much wider – from well below 0·4:1 in Scotland, Ireland and Wales to unity in oriental populations (28). The latter finding illustrates a tendency for the sex ratio in anencephaly to be low if prevalence is high – a tendency which has also sometimes been observed when the sex ratios of anencephalic births in high-risk and low-risk years, social classes, and maternal age and parity groups have been compared (28, 71). However, there are also variations in the prevalence of anencephaly that do *not* seem to be matched by differences in its sex ratio: the east–west gradient in risk across North America, the seasonal trend, and the decline during the last decade (28, 71, 123). Another set of findings suggests that the sex ratio in anencephaly is related to severity: the female preponderance seems to be especially marked in cases in whom rhachischisis, stillbirth and/or early onset hydramnios or labour occur (82, 97, 120, 130).

Twinning. Spina bifida (although not anencephaly) may be less common than average in both monozygotic and dizygotic twins. The evidence comes from data recently assembled by Elwood and Elwood from 24 published series including over 20 000 cases of neural tube defects (28). It is likely that twins were slightly over-represented in these data, since series were included if there were twins among them and excluded if there were not. If this bias is reduced by excluding series of less than 150 cases, and the remaining data are analysed by type of defect, it is found that 2·2% of cases of anencephaly and 1·5% of spina bifida occurred in twins, the figures expected being 2·0% and 2·1% respectively. The difference between the two percentages for anencephaly is not statistically significant, but significantly fewer cases of spina bifida than expected were twins. In the European and North American series for which the sex of each twin pair was recorded, two thirds of the twins with each defect were from like-sexed pairs. As this is similar to the corresponding proportion for all twin pairs of European descent, it does not suggest any difference in prevalence between twins of like- and unlike-sexed pairs or (by inference) between monozygotic and dizygotic twins.

Maternal age and parity. The trends in prevalence with maternal age and parity exhibited by anencephaly and spina bifida are largely similar for the two defects although they differ considerably from place to place. In predominantly Caucasoid countries where the overall prevalence is moderate, such as Canada, the United States and Hungary, the typical trend with each variable is U-shaped. With maternal age, the tendency is for prevalence to decline between teenage pregnancies and those where the mother is in her twenties, but to rise beyond the age of 30 or 35 in each birth rank group. With parity, prevalence generally falls sharply between first and second births in every maternal age group, and increases more gradually from the second or third birth rank upwards, at least when maternal age is high. Longitudinal studies suggest, however, that the average *individual* woman's chance of bearing a child with a neural tube defect lessens in each successive pregnancy, and that the reason why prevalence increases at birth ranks beyond the second or third is that the risks are elevated throughout reproductive life in births to women whose *ultimate* number of pregnancies will be high (who inevitably account for larger proportions of births at higher parities than at lower) (19, 28, 56, 61, 64).

In Great Britain with its higher overall prevalence (at least in the past) the trends observed have been largely similar, with two exceptions: the tendency for first births to be at increased risk has generally been reduced or absent at maternal ages of around 30, and in one large London series no increase at high birth ranks was found (5, 9, 82, 119). During the last few years, however, the upward trend in the prevalence of anencephaly at maternal ages over 35 has disappeared in England and Wales, because the secular decline has been especially marked in this age group (Fig. 1) – perhaps as a result of the increased use of amniocentesis in older women.

The most striking feature of the age-parity pattern in all these countries of moderate or high prevalence is the increased risk among firstborn children. By contrast, in the low-prevalence countries where maternal age and parity effects have been sought (Finland, Israel and Japan), such a primiparity effect seems to be either totally lacking or confined to first births to elderly mothers. Increased risks at high birth ranks, on the other hand, appear to be a feature of low-risk as well as high-risk countries. In Japan, the latter trend in the prevalence of anencephaly seems to be particularly marked at low maternal ages (50, 51, 63, 105).

The above findings imply that the variation in prevalence of neural tube defects between countries is more marked among first births than among later births. The same may be true of their variation over time (28).

Socioeconomic status. Studies of the prevalence of neural tube defects in relation to various indices of socioeconomic status – occupational class of father, locality and quality of home, and type of hospital accommodation at birth – suggest that these defects are relatively rare in the more privileged families, at least in the British Isles, North America and Taiwan (e.g. 5, 15, 22, 29, 37, 61, 107, 154). However, like the associations of prevalence with time, place and personal characteristics that have already been described, the trend with social circumstances seems to vary. For example, the gradient across the Registrar-General's five social classes in the United Kingdom during the 1960s varied according to locality from a fourfold increase extending over all five classes (154) to an increase of less than double between Classes I–II and III–V with little variation within the latter group (9, 25, 85, 91); and no increase at all was detected in Hungary, or among Jews in either Israel or America (19, 105, 107). British and Finnish data suggest that illegitimacy does not add to the risks and may even reduce them, despite its associations with social disadvantage, teenage pregnancy and primiparity (22, 35, 50, 120).

Family history. The last personal characteristics to be considered are aspects of the medical history of family members. Not only have neural tube defects an especially high prevalence in the relatives of persons who have themselves been born with such a defect; they also seem to be commoner than average in the offspring of consanguineous matings (at least in high prevalence areas) (8, 104, 142), and in children born into families with a history of various health problems including miscarriage, stillbirth and child death (20, 28, 46, 50, 93, 121, 125), vertebral anomalies (especially spina bifida occulta) and spinal dysraphism (10, 47, 73, 89, 155), hydrocephaly alone (17), oesophageal atresia (44) and germ cell tumours (3).

Some of the excess miscarriages, stillbirths and child deaths in the sibs of children with neural tube defects are themselves caused by neural tube defects, and thus reflect the tendency for these defects to recur. The excess of stillbirths and child deaths seems to be too great to be entirely explained in this way, but another consideration is that some excess of stillbirths and child deaths among the sibs of children with neural tube defects is to be expected because all these outcomes of pregnancy are especially common in families of low socio-economic status (28). Most analyses of the excess of miscarriages, although not all, suggest that it is maximal in pregnancies immediately preceding those in which neural tube defects occur (14, 40, 77, 93, 121).

Both anencephaly and spina bifida are commoner than average in the relatives of children with either condition, although more often than not when two sibs are affected the second seems to have the same defect as the first (28). The risks quoted below are for defects of either kind occurring in the relatives of children with either.

Data concerning the frequency of neural tube defects in twins of affected infants in 19 series are summarized in Table 2. By Weinberg's method – i.e. by assuming that there were as many dizygotic pairs among the like-sexed as

Table 2. Distribution of twin pairs in which neural tube defects occurred.

Source	No. of discordant pairs		No. of concordant pairs		Prevalence of neural tube defects (per 1000 total births) in related population[b]
	Like-sexed	Unlike-sexed	Like-sexed	Unlike-sexed	
Elwood and Elwood (28)[a]	131	67	11	3	2·9[c]
Record and McKeown (122)	35	14	0	0	4·8 (120)
Fogel et al. (43)	2	1	0	0	1·4 (57)
Field and Kerr (39)	22	9	4	0	2·0 (38)
Myrianthopoulos (102)	4	1	0	0	1·4 (57)
Naggan (106)	13	5	0	1	1·5 (105)
Janerich and Piper (68)	41	14	4	0	1·3 (67)
Buckley and Erten (4)	0	1	1	0	2·6 (4)
Total	248	112	20	4	2·7[c]

[a] Pooled data from 12 reports which gave separately the numbers of neural tube defects of all types observed in like-sexed and unlike-sexed pairs of twins and in the related population. [b] Numbers in brackets refer to the sources from which estimates of prevalence were obtained. [c] Prevalence estimate for pooled populations, weighted according to number of affected twin pairs in each.

among the unlike-sexed – it can be estimated that 232 of the 384 pairs listed were dizygotic and 152 were monozygotic, and that 8 of the former and 16 of the latter pairs were concordant for neural tube defects, i.e. that 19% of the monozygotic twins and 7% of the dizygotic twins of affected individuals were also affected. However, these data have features which suggest that they should be treated with reserve. Three-quarters of the concordant pairs, and only 45% of the discordant, came from just three series based on birth and death registrations; and having seen a non-malformed stillbirth registered as due to anencephaly because a co-twin was so affected, one wonders whether similar events may have caused some discordant pairs in these three series to be counted as concordant.

The prevalence of neural tube defects in nine series of sibs of affected individuals and in the populations to which these individuals belonged is compared in Fig. 2. The data are taken from studies in which diagnoses in

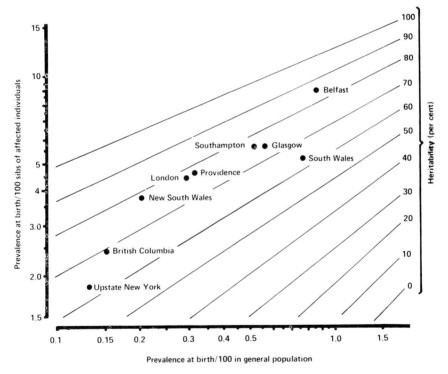

Fig. 2. Prevalence of neural tube defects in nine series of sibs of affected individuals and in the populations to which these individuals belonged. Diagonal lines show the relationship of incidence in first degree relatives to population incidence for various heritability values (135).

relatives were verified from hospital or other records (8, 9, 38, 68, 92, 111, 126, 145, 152, 156). Prevalence in the sibs of cases tends to rise with population prevalence, but the ratio of the former to the latter figure falls from about 15:1 where less than 0·5% of the general population is affected to less than 11:1 where the population prevalence is greater. Prevalence in sibs has also been reported to vary in the same direction as overall prevalence between different social classes (112) and time periods (156).

Among children studied by the authors whose data are represented in Fig. 2, 449 were stated to have been born into sibships where two cases of neural tube defects had already occurred (8, 9, 38, 92, 110, 126, 152, 156). Among these 449 children, 53 (12%) were affected, which is 2·1 times the number that would have been observed if prevalence had been the same in this subgroup of each series as among all the sibs of cases in the same series.

Several of these series also included data for other relatives of cases. When pooled these data yield estimates of prevalence that are higher for maternal than for paternal half-sibs (2·7% and 0·6% respectively) and higher for mothers' sisters' children (9/1000) than for other cousins (4·5/1000). Prevalence among the children of affected parents is about 4·5% regardless of which parent is affected, according to pooled data from three small series (7).

Interpretation of Trends in Prevalence with Demographic Variables

The prevalence of a malformation at birth may vary as a result of variations either in incidence or in the miscarriage rate among affected pregnancies. Two approaches have been used, although only to a limited extent, to explore the importance of miscarriages in this context. The more direct is to see whether any variation in prevalence that has been observed is matched by a variation in incidence as estimated by one of the methods exemplified by Table 1 (p. 157). Virtually the only data so far available that are amenable to this direct approach are those shown in the above table, which suggest that it is because of a difference in miscarriage rates that spina bifida is much less common in Mongoloid than in Caucasoid infants, but that variations in incidence are responsible for the other prevalence trends illustrated – those for both defects within the United Kingdom, and for anencephaly between there and Japan.

The alternative and less direct approach is to assume that if the miscarriage rate among cases of neural tube defects were to vary between different demographic categories of pregnancies, any categories in which this rate was particularly high would also tend to have a high overall miscarriage rate (141). In this case the latter rate would be inversely correlated with any trend in birth prevalence that was due to a variation in the frequency with which affected pregnancies miscarried. Only for two trends in prevalence – the decline between first and second births and the variation between different parts of Great Britain – have opposite trends in the miscarriage rate been reported (36, 128, 141), and this evidence that the geographical trend in the British Isles is due to variation in the miscarriage rate must be weighed against the contrary evidence provided by the more direct approach described above. Among other correlates of the prevalence of neural tube defects, social class has been reported not to be related to the miscarriage rate (128); and there is evidence that high maternal age and conception in spring, like a family history of neural tube defect, are *directly* related to the risks of miscarriage as well as of an affected child being born (86, 94, 141). It therefore seems that trends in incidence brought about by aetiological influences are more likely than variations in miscarriage rates to be responsible for the association between the prevalence of neural tube defects and at least some demographic factors – season of conception, maternal age and socioeconomic status, family history, and (although perhaps only in part) place.

It seems blatantly obvious that the aetiological influences concerned must include both the genotype and other factors – the genotype because of its role in directing embryogenesis and because of the sex difference in liability to neural tube defects, and other factors because of the evidence that these defects occur discordantly in monozygotic twins and that their frequency can vary over time and space in populations of apparently similar genetic composition. Two models of how genetic and other factors might interact to produce such findings have received considerable attention in recent years. First, there is the standard multifactorial model, under which it is assumed that many genetic and environmental factors affect neural tube development; that in each individual embryo these effects can be pictured as adding up to a score; that embryos are normally distributed in respect of these scores; and that neural tube defects occur in embryos whose scores exceed a critical threshold level (151). Second, there is the zygote interaction model, which postulates that neural tube defects occur when the tissues of two zygotes meet in the uterus and interact (69, 71).

The standard multifactorial model. Six predictions of this model have been widely quoted (6), and the above-mentioned data from family studies of neural tube defects appear broadly to satisfy four of them. Firstly, the gradient of risk according to family relationship falls steeply at first and then much more gradually as one passes from monozygotic twins through first-degree and more remote relatives to the general population. Secondly, in high-prevalence populations the tendency is for the risk to sibs to be higher, but for the ratio between this risk and the population prevalence to be lower, than in low-prevalence populations. Thirdly, after two affected births have occurred in a sibship, the risk to subsequent children is higher than after one. Fourthly, prevalence is higher than average in the offspring of consanguineous matings.

The other two predictions are that the relatives of affected males, and of individuals whose defects are more severe than average, should be at higher risk of defects than the relatives of other cases. The prediction that severity and familial prevalence should be associated still needs to be tested – e.g. by making familial comparisons between cases of craniorrhachischisis and of anencephaly with the spine intact: little can be learnt by comparing the risks to relatives of anencephalics and of children with spina bifida (risks which seem to be similar (28)), since the essential difference between the initial errors in development that produce these defects is one of location rather than of degree. The prediction of an especially high risk to the relatives of affected males appears to be false: pooling the data from those of the above-quoted series in which the sibs of male and female cases were analysed separately (8, 9, 38, 111, 126, 152) yields figures for the prevalence of neural tube defects in these two groups which are virtually identical – 5·2% and 5·1% respectively. However, the contrasts between children of these kinds predicted by the multifactorial model, e.g. a ratio of 1·14:1 between the risks to children born after an affected male and after an affected female in a community where prevalence in males was 0·56 times that in females (72), are not so great as to warrant a complete rejection of the model, given its consistency with most of the familial data.

One appealing feature of this model is that at first sight it seems to provide a way of quantifying the relative contributions made by genetic and other influences to the causation of any defect to which it applies. To be more precise, given the defect's incidence in the general population and in any one class of relatives, we can calculate its *heritability* – the proportion that genetic factors could be contributing to the variance of the scores that determine which individuals are affected. In Fig. 2 (p. 165), the diagonal lines show the relationship between incidence in first degree relatives and population incidence for various heritability values. They indicate that if the family study data plotted in Fig. 2 had been incidence statistics, the corresponding heritability values would have been between 63% and 85%. In the same circumstances the estimated risks given on p. 165 for monozygotic and dizygotic twins of cases would correspond to heritability values of about 70% and 95% respectively – although the last of these values must be viewed with particular reserve, in view of the small numbers on which it is based.

However, there are two general problems about estimating heritability in this way – firstly that data on prevalence at birth have been used instead of incidence data, and secondly that the method treats as heritable not only the effects of the genotype but also those of any environmental influences on frequency that tend to be shared by relatives. Where incidence is higher than prevalence, the use of prevalence data introduces a downward bias: thus, even if the incidence in each of the populations and groups of sibs examined in Fig. 2 had been higher than prevalence by only 50% (a conservative estimate), the incidence data would have yielded heritability values of 68–97% instead of the values of 63–85% based on prevalence. The sharing of environmental factors by relatives, on the other hand, introduces an upward bias into heritability values. Factors of this kind are particularly likely to be shared by children who develop in the same uterus or in the uteri of related women. The view that such factors are involved in the aetiology of neural tube defects is therefore supported by the evidence that the prevalence of neural tube defects among the relatives of affected children is higher in half-sibs with the same mother than in those with the same father, and higher in cousins whose mothers are sisters than in other cousins (p. 166). However, these differences may also be due at least in part to the mothers of cases – the usual informants in family studies – being most fully informed about their own and their sisters' children.

Given so many uncertainties, it seems that although the standard multifactorial model may be broadly applicable to neural tube defects, little reliance should be placed upon the heritability values that it yields.

The zygote interaction model. This model was proposed by Knox (69, 71), who postulated that interaction might occur if an embryo with certain gene-based recognition factors – characteristics involved in the process by which the tissues of mother and embryo recognize each other – was to encounter tissues from a zygote in which one or more of these factors was lacking. This second zygote might be either a dizygotic twin or other litter mate of the first, or the product of a previous conception from which some trophoblast had remained in the uterus. The interaction was envisaged as causing malformation of the first zygote and elimination of the second. Knox showed that if the genes controlling at least one set of recognition factors were sex-linked, any malformation that occurred in the embryos that survived interaction would be likely to show several of the features which appeared to be characteristic of neural tube defects – a low rate of concordance in twins, a tendency to affect more females than males and more twins from like-sexed pairs than from unlike-sexed, and a prevalence in the sibs of cases which is several times as high as in the general population but low enough for the great majority to be unaffected. If in addition the zygotes that could interact did not do so in every instance, but only in a proportion that was affected by environmental factors, Knox also noted that the excess of females among the malformed would tend either not to change with variations in prevalence of environmental origin or to be directly correlated with them, depending on whether interaction could be precipitated by the products of only one or of more than one allele at the sex-linked locus that he envisaged. This could explain why there should be some evidence of a direct association between prevalence and the extent of the female preponderance in anencephaly but not in spina bifida (p. 161). Another epidemiological finding for which this model provides an explanation is the evidence that pregnancies that occur next after ones that have miscarried are at increased risk of neural tube defects (p. 163). It seems that most chorionepitheliomata (malignant neoplasms of trophoblast) occur after abortive and molar pregnancies, which suggests that trophoblastic tissue is more often left in the uterus by aborted zygotes and hydatidiform moles than by offspring who survive (14).

Arguments against zygote interaction being the major cause of neural tube defects include firstly the relatively high prevalence of these in groups such as firstborn children in which the proportion that has been exposed to tissue from other zygotes is unlikely to be increased (32); secondly the failure of several studies to demonstrate any tendency for affected infants to be conceived after an inter-pregnancy interval of longer or shorter than average duration (14, 21, 77); and thirdly the fact that the concordance rate in twins with neural tube defects seems from recently published data (Table 2, p. 164) to be considerably higher than the figure considered by Knox which the model seemed to fit. However, although these considerations suggest that at best the model is incomplete (as Knox himself said when he first presented it), they do not exclude the possibility that some kind of zygote interaction is involved in the aetiology of neural tube defects.

Specific Causes of Neural Tube Defects

Although both the zygote interaction model and the standard multifactorial model suggest that environmental as well as genetic influences are involved in the causation of neural tube defects, the only specific environmental influence that is envisaged by either model is the tissue, from a zygote other than the one at risk, on which the zygote interaction model focuses. The other non-genetic factors that human studies suggest that we should seriously consider as causes of neural tube defects have largely been identified by clinical observation, by attempts to correlate the differences in prevalence that exist between demographic groups with variations in the exposure of these groups to possible causes, and by retrospective case-control studies, occasionally followed by prospective studies of cohorts of pregnant women and/or by intervention studies.

The factors of greatest current interest are of course nutritional. Other contributors to this workshop have fully discussed recent work in this field.

For this reason it will not be reviewed here, except to make the point that it illustrates admirably how aetiological research can be furthered by a combination of all the kinds of studies in humans just mentioned, as well as by work with laboratory animals. The hypothesis that nutritional deficiencies might be involved in causing human neural tube defects was first made to appear attractive by studies of three kinds: firstly the animal experiments of Hale (53), Warkany (150), Giroud (49) and their successors, in which neural tube defects and other malformations were produced by vitamin deficiencies; secondly the clinical observation of Thiersch (143, 144), who reported neural tube defects in the offspring of women who had been given aminopterin, a folate antagonist, to test its efficacy as an abortifacient; and thirdly the descriptive studies of the prevalence of neural tube defects in humans (pp. 157–166), which suggested a link with nutrition by revealing variations with season and social class. At least four methods have subsequently been used to test this hypothesis in human populations:

(1) The extent to which the variations in prevalence between different groups are correlated with nutritional differences has been explored, in surveys in which the diet and nutrition of women in early pregnancy in Leeds (136, 137) and London (see p. 197) were observed and comparisons made between the high-risk and low-risk social classes and (in the London study) seasons. The women in the low-risk classes (social classes I and II) had the higher dietary and blood vitamin levels. Mean blood folate levels were lowest in the women examined in spring, the time when the children at highest seasonal risk are conceived.

(2) The retrospective case-control method was used by Laurence's group (75) when they questioned mothers of affected children in south Wales about their diets during every pregnancy, with results which suggested that diets were on average poorer during the affected pregnancies than during the others. Another case-control design, in which mothers whose children had malformations of the central nervous system were matched with mothers of unaffected children, was used by Hibbard and Smithells (58) in a study which suggested that folate deficiency at the end of pregnancy, as detected by the formimino-glutamic acid excretion test, was particularly common in the former group.

(3) Prospective cohort study methods were also used in the above-mentioned surveys in Leeds and south Wales, in that women whose nutritional state had been assessed in early pregnancy were followed up to see whether this was correlated with the outcome of the same pregnancy. Among the women who then produced affected offspring,

those in the Leeds study were found to have relatively low mean red cell folate and white cell vitamin C levels (137) and those in South Wales were all among the 24% of women in the study whose diet during the first trimester had been classified as poor (74, 75).

(4) Intervention studies have been carried out by Laurence, Smithells and their colleagues in women who had previously borne at least one child with a neural tube defect and who wished to become pregnant again. With each of the interventions used – dietary counselling (75), folate (76) and a multivitamin and iron preparation (138, 139) – a smaller proportion of the treated women's offspring had neural tube defects than of those with whom they were compared.

There are of course various criticisms that can be directed against aspects of this work. For example, the information on diet in pregnancy furnished by the mothers in the South Wales studies was not very precise, and was in part collected retrospectively when it could have been biased by the mothers' knowledge of the outcome of pregnancy; and of the intervention studies, one used controls that were not randomized, and in the others the differences in neural tube defect frequency between the controls and the women who were allocated treatment were not statistically significant. It is nevertheless impressive to find so great a degree of consistency between the results of studies of so many kinds.

The nutritional problem for which these studies provide most evidence of a causal relationship to neural tube defects is folate deficiency. Interest was also aroused in the fairly recent past by reports of correlations, particularly in space and time, between the prevalence of these defects and the uptake of various other constituents of food and drink – inverse correlations of prevalence with the total hardness or magnesium or calcium content of drinking water (26, 33, 91, 149), and direct correlations with consumption of tea (34), potatoes affected by blight (124), nitrates and nitrites in cured meats, and magnesium salts in canned peas (70). Other considerations suggest however that most of these associations are not causal. The magnesium ion seems unlikely to have opposite effects depending on its source. Negative findings have emerged from various studies designed to test whether the prevalence of defects is correlated with potato blight (28), cured meat intake (25) or electrolyte levels (27, 100, 101) in data sets other than those in which such correlations were originally found. Largely negative results were also obtained in case-control comparisons of potato consumption (28) and of electrolytes in drinking water (131), and in cohort studies of women who abstained from potatoes during pregnancy having previously borne affected children (28). Tea-drinking and below-average amounts of zinc in drinking water seem to be the only factors for which the case-control studies prompted by the above correlations have provided any evidence of a relationship to neural tube defects; and each of these two factors only seems to have been examined in one case-control study (34, 131). However, the finding for zinc accords with the evidence that serum and red cell zinc levels tend to be lower than average in women whose offspring have malformations (including neural tube defects) and possibly in the affected offspring as well (11, 12, 66, 140) and that zinc deficiency causes neural tube defects in rats (62) and occurs in areas of the Middle East where anencephaly is relatively common (133).

Apart from diet-related factors, the main groups of environmental influences that have been explored as possible causes of neural tube defects (as indeed of other malformations) are drugs and diseases. However, there seems to be little evidence for the production of neural tube defects in humans by any drug apart from those that cause folate depletion, or by any specific maternal disease with the exception of diabetes – in which neural tube defects account for a substantial part of the overall excess of malformations (84). Several case-control and cohort studies suggest that neural tube defects are also commoner than average in children whose mothers were affected during early pregnancy by influenza or by other causes of hyperthermia (13, 16, 28, 41, 51, 54, 78, 153), but there is also evidence that the prevalence of these defects is not especially high in children whose embryonic development has occurred in places and periods in which influenza or sauna-bathing (which also induces hyperthermia) has been widespread (79, 81, 118). These two sets of findings may perhaps be reconciled by postulating that the risk to the embryo is not increased by febrile conditions of the mother *per se*, but rather by some feature of mothers whose resistance to infection is low.

It may be concluded that what we know about the specific causes of neural tube defects in humans is still very limited, but that besides being high for the offspring of diabetics the risks are probably increased by folate deficiency and possibly by zinc deficiency. Among the evidence for this view, the biochemical data on folate and zinc levels hold an important place, and suggest that other biochemical comparisons between affected and normal offspring and their mothers might be revealing and should be given high priority in future research. When such comparisons are made at the time of birth, it may sometimes be difficult to distinguish abnormal values that are secondary to the malformation from ones that are primary; but maternal abnormalities of the latter kind may tend to persist, and be identifiable by comparing the mothers of cases and controls at a later stage. The ideal time to do this might be during subsequent pregnancies, but for some relevant substances (notably red cell folate), quite high correlations have even been observed between maternal levels in early pregnancy and in the non-pregnant state one year later (see p. 197).

The levels, in blood and other tissues, of the nutrients, electrolytes or other substances that influence development must of course be influenced not only by intake but also by constitutional factors. It therefore seems likely that at least part of the influence of the genotype on the risk of malformation is mediated through its effects on tissue levels that may also be affected by diet and other variables in the environment, in which case it should be possible to overcome the adverse effects of a high-risk genotype by manipulating these variables. This could be one reason for the low recurrence rates observed by Laurence, Smithells and their colleagues after giving periconceptional vitamin supplements and dietary advice to women who had previously borne affected children.

References

1. Baird, D. (1980). Environment and reproduction. *Brit. J. Obstet. Gynaecol.* **87**, 1057–1067.
2. Biggar, R. J., Mortimer, E. A. and Haughie, G. E. (1976). Descriptive epidemiology of neural tube defects, Rochester, New York, 1918–1938. *Am. J. Epidemiol.* **104**, 22–27.
3. Birch, J. M. (1980). Anencephaly in stillborn sibs of children with germ cell tumours. *Lancet* **i**, 1257.
4. Buckley, M. R. and Erten, O. (1979). The epidemiology of anencephaly and spina bifida in Izmir, Turkey, in the light of recent epidemiological theories. *J. Epidemiol. Comm. Health* **33**, 186–190.
5. Butler, N. R., Alberman, E. D. and Schutt, W. H. (1969). The congenital malformations. *In* "Perinatal Problems" (Second Report of the British Perinatal Mortality Survey) (N. R. Butler and E. D. Alberman, eds) pp. 283–320. Livingstone, Edinburgh.
6. Carter, C. O. (1969). Genetics of common disorders. *Brit. Med. Bull.* **25**, 52–57.
7. Carter, C. O. (1976). Genetics of common single malformations. *Brit. Med. Bull.* **32**, 21–26.
8. Carter, C. O., David, P. A. and Laurence, K. M. (1968). A family study of major central nervous system malformations in South Wales. *J. Med. Genet.* **5**, 81–106.
9. Carter, C. O. and Evans, K. A. (1973). Spina bifida and anencephalus in Greater London. *J. Med. Genet.* **10**, 209–234.
10. Carter, C. O., Evans, K. A. and Till, K. (1976). Congenital scoliosis caused by multiple defects of the vertebral bodies. *J. Med. Genet.* **13**, 343–350.
11. Çavdar, A. O. (1982). Zinc and small babies. *Lancet* **i**, 339–340.
12. Çavdar, A. O., Arcasoy, A., Baycu, T. and Himmetoglu, O. (1980). Zinc deficiency and anencephaly in Turkey. *Teratology* **22**, 141.
13. Chance, P. F. and Smith, D. W. (1978). Hyperthermia and meningomyelocele and anencephaly. *Lancet* **i**, 769–770.
14. Clarke, C., Hobson, D., McKendrick, O. M., Rogers, S. C. and Sheppard, P. M. (1975). Spina bifida and anencephaly: miscarriage as possible cause. *Brit. Med. J.* **iv**, 743–746.

15. Coffey, V. P. and Jessop, W. J. E. (1957). A study of 137 cases of anencephaly. *Brit. J. Prev. Soc. Med.* 11, 174–180.
16. Coffey, V. P. and Jessop, W. J. E. (1963). Maternal influenza and congenital deformities. A follow-up study. *Lancet* i, 748–751.
17. Cohen, T., Stern, E. and Rosenmann, A. (1979). Sib risk of neural tube defect: is prenatal diagnosis indicated in pregnancies following the birth of a hydrocephalic child? *J. Med. Genet.* 16, 14–16.
18. Creasy, M. R. and Alberman, E. D. (1976). Congenital malformations of the central nervous system in spontaneous abortions. *J. Med. Genet.* 13, 9–16.
19. Czeizel, A. and Révész, C. (1970). Major malformations of the central nervous system in Hungary. *Brit. J. Prev. Soc. Med.* 24, 205–222.
20. David, T. J. and Smith, C. M. (1980). Outcome of pregnancy after spontaneous abortion. *Brit. Med. J.* 280, 447–448.
21. Durkin, M. V., Kaveggia, E. G., Pendleton, E. and Opitz, J. M. (1976). Sequential fetus-fetus interaction and CNS defects. *Lancet* ii, 43.
22. Edwards, J. H. (1958). Congenital malformations of the central nervous system in Scotland. *Brit. J. Prev. Soc. Med.* 12, 115–130.
23. Eichmann, E. and Gesenius, H. (1952). Die Missgeburtenzunahme in Berlin und Umgebung in den Nachkriegsjahren. *Archiv für Gynaekologie* 181, 168–184.
24. Elwood, J. H. (1970). Anencephalus in Belfast: incidence and secular and seasonal variations, 1950–66. *Brit. J. Prev. Soc. Med.* 24, 78–88.
25. Elwood, J. H. and Nevin, N. C. (1973). Factors associated with anencephalus and spina bifida in Belfast. *Brit. J. Prev. Soc. Med.* 27, 73–80.
26. Elwood, J. M. (1977). Anencephalus and drinking water composition. *Am. J. Epidemiol.* 105, 460–467.
27. Elwood, J. M. and Coldman, A. J. (1981). Water composition in the etiology of anencephalus. *Am. J. Epidemiol.* 113, 681–690.
28. Elwood, J. M. and Elwood, J. H. (1980). "Epidemiology of Anencephalus and Spina Bifida." Oxford University Press, Oxford.
29. Emanuel, I., Huang, S.-W., Gutman, L. T., Yu, F.-C. and Lin, C.-C. (1972). The incidence of congenital malformations in a Chinese population. *Teratology* 5, 159–170.
30. Emanuel, I. and Sever, L. E. (1973). Questions concerning the possible association of potatoes and neural tube defects, and an alternative hypothesis relating to maternal growth and development. *Teratology* 8, 325–331.
31. Erickson, J. D. (1976). Racial variations in the incidence of congenital malformations. *Ann. Human Genet.* 39, 315–320.
32. Evans, D. R. (1979). Neural tube defects: importance of a history of abortion in aetiology. *Brit. Med. J.* i, 975–976.
33. Fedrick, J. (1970). Anencephalus and the local water supply. *Nature* 227, 176–177.
34. Fedrick, J. (1974). Anencephalus and maternal tea drinking: evidence for a possible association. *Proc. Roy. Soc. Med.* 67, 356–360.
35. Fedrick, J. (1976). Anencephalus in the Oxford Record Linkage Study Area. *Dev. Med. Child Neurol.* 18, 643–656.
36. Fedrick, J. and Adelstein, P. (1976). Area differences in the incidence of neural tube defect and the rate of spontaneous abortion. *Brit. J. Prev. Soc. Med.* 30, 32–35.
37. Feldman, J. G., Stein, S. C., Klein, R. J., Kohl, S. and Casey, G. (1982). The

prevalence of neural tube defects among ethnic groups in Brooklyn, New York. *J. Chron. Dis.* **35**, 53–60.
38. Field, B. (1978). Neural tube defects in New South Wales, Australia. *J. Med. Genet.* **15**, 329–338.
39. Field, B. and Kerr, C. (1974). Twinning and neural-tube defects. *Lancet* **ii**, 964–965.
40. Field, B. and Kerr, C. (1976). Aetiology of anencephaly and spina bifida. *Brit. Med. J.* **iii**, 107.
41. Fisher, N. L. and Smith, D. W. (1981). Occipital encephalocele and early gestational hyperthermia. *Pediatrics* **68**, 480–483.
42. Fishman, M. A., Maedjono, S. J. and Taysi, K. (1978). Normal karyotypes in infants with neural-tube defects. *New Eng. J. Med.* **298**, 1149–1150.
43. Fogel, B. J., Nitowsky, H. M. and Greunwald, P. (1965). Discordant abnormalities in monozygotic twins. *J. Pediatrics* **66**, 64–72.
44. Fraser, F. C. and Nussbaum, E. (1980). Neural tube defects in children with tracheo-oesophageal dysraphism. *Lancet* **ii**, 807.
45. French, F. E. and Bierman, J. M. (1962). Probabilities of fetal mortality. *Public Health Reports (Washington)* **77**, 835–847.
46. Gardiner, A., Clarke, C., Cowen, J., Finn, R. and McKendrick, O. M. (1978). Spontaneous abortion and fetal abnormality in subsequent pregnancy. *Brit. Med. J.* **i**, 1016–1018.
47. Gardner, R. J. M., Alexander, C. and Veale, A. M. O. (1974). Spina bifida occulta in the parents of offspring with neural tube defects. *Journal de Génétique Humaine* **22**, 389–395.
48. Ghosh, A., Woo, J. S. K., Poon, I. M. L. and Ma, H.-K. (1981). Neural-tube defects in Hong Kong Chinese. *Lancet* **ii**, 468–469.
49. Giroud, A. (1955). Les malformations congénitales et leurs causes. *Biologie Médicale* **44**, 1–86.
50. Granroth, G., Haapakoski, J. and Hakama, M. (1978). Defects of the central nervous system in Finland: II. Birth order, outcome of previous pregnancies and family history. *Teratology* **17**, 213–222.
51. Granroth, G., Haapakoski, J. and Saxén, L. (1978). Defects of the central nervous system in Finland: V. Multivariate analysis of risk indicators. *Int. J. Epidemiol.* **7**, 301–308.
52. Granroth, G., Hakama, M. and Saxén, L. (1977). Defects of the central nervous system in Finland: I. Variations in time and space, sex distribution, and parental age. *Brit. J. Prev. Soc. Med.* **31**, 164–170.
53. Hale, F. (1935). The relation of vitamin A to anophthalmos in pigs. *Am. J. Ophthalmol.* **18**, 1087–1092.
54. Halperin, L. R. and Wilroy, R. S. (1978). Maternal hyperthermia and neural-tube defects. *Lancet* **ii**, 212–213.
55. Harris, M. J. and Poland, B. J. (1978). Neural tube defects in human spontaneous abortuses: diagnosis and relevance to counselling. *Teratology* **17**, 28A.
56. Hay, S. and Barbano, H. (1972). Independent effects of maternal age and birth order on the incidence of selected congenital malformations. *Teratology* **6**, 271–279.
57. Heinonen, O. P., Slone, D. and Shapiro, S. (1977). "Birth Defects and Drugs in Pregnancy." Publishing Sciences Group, Littleton, Mass.
58. Hibbard, E. D. and Smithells, R. W. (1965). Folic acid metabolism and human embryopathy. *Lancet* **i**, 1254.

59. Hobbs, M. S. T. (1969). Risk of anencephaly in migrant and non-migrant women in the Oxford Area. *Brit. J. Prev. Soc. Med.* **23**, 174–178.

60. Hook, E. B., Albright, S. G. and Cross, P. K. (1980). Use of Bernoulli Census and log-linear methods for estimating the prevalence of spina bifida in live births and the completeness of vital record reports in New York State. *Am. J. Epidemiol.* **112**, 750–758.

61. Horowitz, I. and McDonald, A. D. (1969). Anencephaly and spina bifida in the Province of Quebec. *Can. Med. Assoc. J.* **100**, 748–755.

62. Hurley, L. S. and Schrader, R. E. (1972). Congenital malformations of the nervous system in zinc deficient rats. *In* "Neurobiology of the Trace Metals Zinc and Copper" (C. C. Pfeiffer, ed.), pp. 7–51. Academic Press, London and New York.

63. Imaizumi, Y. (1979). Anencephaly in Japan: paternal age, maternal age and birth order. *Ann. Human Genet.* **42**, 445–455.

64. Ingalls, T. H., Pugh, T. F. and MacMahon, B. (1954). Incidence of anencephalus, spina bifida and hydrocephalus related to birth rank and maternal age. *Brit. J. Prev. Soc. Med.* **8**, 17–23.

65. James, L. M. and Erickson, J. D. (1979). Anencephaly and spina bifida: high rates in Appalachia? *Am. J. Human Genet.* **31**, 136A.

66. Jameson, S. (1976). Variations in maternal serum zinc during pregnancy and correlation to congenital malformations, dysmaturity, and abnormal parturition. *Acta Medica Scandinavica*, suppl. **593**, 21–37.

67. Janerich, D. T. (1973). Epidemic waves in the prevalence of anencephaly and spina bifida in New York State. *Teratology* **8**, 253–256.

68. Janerich, D. T. and Piper, J. (1978). Shifting genetic patterns in anencephaly and spina bifida. *J. Med. Genet.* **15**, 101–105.

69. Knox, E. G. (1970). Fetus-fetus interaction – a model aetiology for anencephalus. *Dev. Med. Child Neurol.* **12**, 167–177.

70. Knox, E. G. (1972). Anencephalus and dietary intakes. *Brit. J. Prev. Soc. Med.* **26**, 219–223.

71. Knox, E. G. (1974). Twins and neural tube defects. *Brit. J. Prev. Soc. Med.* **28**, 73–80.

72. Lalouel, J. M., Morton, N. E. and Jackson, J. (1979). Neural tube malformations: complex segregation analysis and calculation of recurrence risk. *J. Med. Genet.* **16**, 8–13.

73. Laurence, K. M. (1970). Vertebral abnormalities in first degree relatives of cases of spina bifida and of anencephaly. *Arch. Dis. Child.* **45**, 274.

74. Laurence, K. M. (1982). The role of improvement in the maternal diet and preconceptional folic acid supplementation in the prevention of neural tube defects. This volume, pp. 85–108.

75. Laurence, K. M., James, N., Miller, M. and Campbell, H. (1980). Increased risk of recurrence of pregnancies complicated by fetal neural tube defects in mothers receiving poor diets, and possible benefit of dietary counselling. *Brit. Med. J.* **281**, 1592–1594.

76. Laurence, K. M., James, N., Miller, M. H., Tennant, G. B. and Campbell, H. (1981). Double-blind randomised controlled trial of folate treatment before conception to prevent recurrence of neural-tube defects. *Brit. Med. J.* **282**, 1509–1511.

77. Laurence, K. M. and Roberts, C. J. (1977). Spina bifida and anencephaly: are miscarriages a possible cause? *Brit. Med. J.* **ii**, 361–362.
78. Layde, P. M., Edmonds, L. D. and Erickson, J. D. (1980). Maternal fever and neural tube defects. *Teratology* **21**, 105–108.
79. Leck, I. (1963). Incidence of malformations following influenza epidemics. *Brit. J. Prev. Soc. Med.* **17**, 70–80.
80. Leck, I. (1966). Changes in the incidence of neural tube defects. *Lancet* **ii**, 791–793.
81. Leck, I. (1971). Further tests of the hypothesis that influenza in pregnancy causes malformations. *H.S.M.H.A. Health Reports* **86**, 265–269.
82. Leck, I. (1972). The etiology of human malformations: insights from epidemiology. *Teratology* **5**, 303–314.
83. Leck, I. (1977). Correlations of malformation frequency with environmental and genetic attributes in man. *In* "Handbook of Teratology", Vol. 3 (Comparative, Maternal and Epidemiological Aspects) (J. G. Wilson and F. C. Fraser, eds) pp. 234–324. Plenum, New York.
84. Leck, I. (1979). Teratogenic risks of disease and therapy. *In* "Epidemiologic Methods for Detection of Teratogens" (Contributions to Epidemiology and Biostatistics, vol. 1) (M. A. Klingberg and J. A. C. Weatherall, eds) pp. 23–43. Karger, Basle.
85. Leck, I. (1981). Epidemiological aspects of paediatrics: insights into the causation of disorders of early life. *In* "Scientific Foundations of Paediatrics", 2nd edition (J. A. Davis and J. Dobbing, eds) pp. 947–979. Heinemann, London.
86. Leck, I. and Record, R. G. (1966). Seasonal incidence of anencephalus. *Brit. J. Prev. Soc. Med.* **20**, 67–75.
87. Leck, I. and Rogers, S. C. (1967). Changes in the incidence of anencephalus. *Brit. J. Prev. Soc. Med.* **21**, 177–180.
88. Lesi, F. E. A. (1969). The significance of congenital defects in developing countries. *Med. Today* **3**, 26–40.
89. Lorber, J. and Levick, K. (1967). Spina bifida cystica. Incidence of spina bifida occulta in parents and in controls. *Arch. Dis. Child.* **42**, 171–173.
90. Lowe, C. R. (1972). Congenital malformations and the problem of their control. *Brit. Med. J.* **iii**, 515–520.
91. Lowe, C. R., Roberts, C. L. and Lloyd, S. (1971). Malformations of the central nervous system and softness of local water supplies. *Brit. Med. J.* **ii**, 357–361.
92. McBride, M. L. (1978). Familial risks of anencephaly and spina bifida in British Columbia. M.Sc. thesis, University of British Columbia.
93. McDonald, A. D. (1971). Abortion in neural tube defect fraternities. *Brit. J. Prev. Soc. Med.* **25**, 220–221.
94. McDonald, A. D. (1971). Seasonal distribution of abortions. *Brit. J. Prev. Soc. Med.* **25**, 222–224.
95. MacHenry, J. C. R. M., Nevin, N. C. and Merrett, J. D. (1979). Comparison of central nervous system malformations in spontaneous abortions in Northern Ireland and south-east England. *Brit. Med. J.* **i**, 1395–1397.
96. McKeown, T. and Record, R. G. (1951). Seasonal incidence of congenital malformations of the central nervous system. *Lancet* **i**, 192–196.
97. MacMahon, B. and McKeown, T. (1952). A note on the sex ratio in anencephalus. *Brit. J. Prev. Soc. Med.* **6**, 265–266.
98. MacMahon, B. and Yen, S. (1971). Unrecognised epidemic of anencephaly and spina bifida. *Lancet* **i**, 31–33.

99. MacMahon, B. and Yen, S. (1971). Influenza and neural tube defects. *Lancet* ii, 260–261.
100. Morton, M. S., Elwood, P. C. and Abernethy, M. (1976). Trace elements in water and congenital malformations of the central nervous system in South Wales. *Brit. J. Prev. Soc. Med.* **30**, 36–39.
101. Morton, M. S., Elwood, P. C. and St. Leger, A. S. (1976). Trace elements in water and congenital malformations of the central nervous system. *Teratology* **14**, 368.
102. Myrianthopoulos, N. C. (1975). Congenital malformations in twins: epidemiologic survey. *Birth Defects Original Article Series* 11, No. 8.
103. Myrianthopoulos, N. C. and Chung, C. S. (1974). Congenital malformations in singletons: epidemiologic survey. *Birth Defects Original Article Series* 10, No. 11.
104. Naderi, S. (1979). Congenital abnormalities in newborns of consanguineous and nonconsanguineous parents. *Obstet. Gynecol.* **53**, 195–199.
105. Naggan, L. (1971). Anencephaly and spina bifida in Israel. *Pediatrics* **47**, 577–586.
106. Naggan, L. (1976). I. Methodology of ascertainment in international comparisons. II. Anencephaly and spina bifida in Israel. *In* "Birth Defects: Risks and Consequences" (S. Kelly, E. B. Hook, D. T. Janerich and I. H. Porter, eds) pp. 41–58. Academic Press, New York and London.
107. Naggan, L. and MacMahon, B. (1967). Ethnic differences in the prevalence of anencephaly and spina bifida in Boston, Massachusetts. *New Eng. J. Med.* **277**, 1119–1123.
108. Neel, J. V. (1958). A study of major congenital defects in Japanese infants. *Am. J. Human Genet.* **10**, 398–445.
109. Nevin, N. C. (1982). Prevention of neural tube defects in an area of high incidence. This volume, pp. 127–144.
110. Nevin, N. C. and Johnston, W. P. (1980). Risk of recurrence after two children with central nervous system malformations in an area of high incidence. *J. Med. Genet.* **17**, 87–92.
111. Nevin, N. C. and Johnston, W. P. (1980). A family study of spina bifida and anencephalus in Belfast, Northern Ireland (1964 to 1968). *J. Med. Genet.* **17**, 203–211.
112. Nevin, N. C., Johnston, W. P. and Merrett, J. D. (1981). Influence of social class on the risk of recurrence of anencephalus and spina bifida. *Dev. Med. Child Neurol.* **23**, 155–159.
113. Nishimura, H. (1975). Prenatal versus postnatal malformations based on the Japanese experience on induced abortions in the human being. *In* "Aging Gametes: Their Biology and Pathology" (Proceedings of the International Symposium on Aging Gametes, Seattle, Wash., June 13–16, 1973) (R. J. Blandau, ed.) pp. 349–368. Karger, Basel.
114. Office of Population Censuses and Surveys (1981). OPCS Monitor Reference MB3 81/4: Congenital Malformations. Government Statistical Service, London.
115. Ogbalu, M. M., Leck, I. and Hillier, V. F. (1977). The prevalence of malformations at birth in southern Nigeria. Paper presented at the Fifth International Conference on Birth Defects, Montreal, Canada, August 1977.
116. Owens, J. R., Harris, F., McAllister, E. and West, L. (1981). 19-year incidence of neural tube defects in area under constant surveillance. *Lancet* ii, 1032–1035.

117. Parker, G. (1978). Season of birth in New South Wales. *Med. J. Aust.* **2**, 563–566.
118. Rapola, J., Saxén, K. and Granroth, G. (1978). Anencephaly and the sauna. *Lancet* **i**, 1162.
119. Record, R. G. (1961). Anencephalus in Scotland. *Brit. J. Prev. Soc. Med.* **15**, 93–105.
120. Record, R. G. and McKeown, T. (1949). Congenital malformations of the central nervous system: 1. A survey of 930 cases. *Brit. J. Soc. Med.* **3**, 183–219.
121. Record, R. G. and McKeown, T. (1950). Congenital malformations of the central nervous system. II – Maternal reproductive history and familial incidence. *Brit. J. Soc. Med.* **4**, 26–50.
122. Record, R. G. and McKeown, T. (1951). Congenital malformations of the central nervous system: data on 69 pairs of twins. *Ann. Eugenics* **15**, 285–292.
123. Registrar General (1963–81). Registrar-General's Statistical Reviews of England and Wales for the Years 1961–1974. Part I: Tables, Medical. Mortality Statistics: Childhood (Reviews of the Registrar General on Deaths in England and Wales, 1974–1975: Series DH3, nos 1 and 2). Mortality Statistics: Childhood and Maternity (Reviews of the Registrar General on Deaths in England and Wales, 1976–1979): Series DH3, nos 3–6). Her Majesty's Stationery Office, London.
124. Renwick, J. H. (1972). Hypothesis: anencephaly and spina bifida are usually preventable by avoidance of a specific but unidentified substance present in certain potato tubers. *Brit. J. Prev. Soc. Med.* **26**, 67–88.
125. Richards, I. D. G. (1973). Fetal and infant mortality associated with congenital malformations. *Brit. J. Prev. Soc. Med.* **27**, 85–90.
126. Richards, I. D. G., McIntosh, H. T. and Sweenie, S. (1972). A genetic study of anencephaly and spina bifida in Glasgow. *Dev. Med. Child Neurol.* **14**, 626–639.
127. Richards, I. D. G., Roberts, C. J. and Lloyd, S. (1972). Area differences in prevalence of neural tube malformations in South Wales. A study of possible demographic determinants. *Brit. J. Prev. Soc. Med.* **26**, 89–93.
128. Roberts, C. J. and Lloyd, S. (1973). Area differences in spontaneous abortion rates in South Wales and their relation to neural tube defect incidence. *Brit. Med. J.* **iv**, 20–22.
129. Rogers, S. C. and Weatherall, J. A. C. (1976). Anencephalus, Spina Bifida and Congenital Hydrocephalus: England and Wales, 1964–1972 (Studies on Medical and Population Studies No. 32). Her Majesty's Stationery Office, London.
130. Sagar, H. J. and Desa, D. J. (1973). The relationship between hydramnios and some characteristics of the infant in pregnancies complicated by fetal anencephaly. *J. Obstet. Gynaecol. Brit. Commonwealth* **80**, 429–432.
131. St. Leger, A. S., Elwood, P. C. and Morton, M. S. (1980). Neural tube malformations and trace elements in water. *J. Epidemiol. Community Health* **34**, 186–187.
132. Searle, A. G. (1959). The incidence of anencephaly in a polytypic population. *Ann. Human Genet.* **23**, 279–288.
133. Sever, L. E. and Emanuel, I. (1973). Is there a connection between maternal zinc deficiency and congenital malformations of the central nervous system in man? *Teratology* **7**, 117–118.
134. Slater, B. C. S., Watson, G. I. and McDonald, J. C. (1964). Seasonal variation in congenital abnormalities: preliminary report of a survey conducted by the

Research Committee of Council of the College of General Practitioners. *Brit. J. Prev. Soc. Med.* **18**, 1–7.
135. Smith, C. (1970). Heritability of liability and concordance in monozygous twins. *Ann. Human Genet.* **34**, 85–91.
136. Smithells, R. W., Ankers, C., Carver, M. E., Lennon, D., Schorah, C. J. and Sheppard, S. (1977). Maternal nutrition in early pregnancy. *Brit. J. Nutrition* **38**, 497–506.
137. Smithells, R. W., Sheppard, S. and Schorah, C. J. (1976). Vitamin deficiencies and neural tube defects. *Arch. Dis. Child.* **51**, 944–950.
138. Smithells, R. W., Sheppard, S., Schorah, C. J., Seller, M. J., Nevin, N. C., Harris, R., Read, A. P. and Fielding, D. W. (1981). Apparent prevention of neural tube defects by vitamin supplementation. *Arch. Dis. Child.* **56**, 911–918.
139. Smithells, R. W., Sheppard, S., Schorah, C. J., Seller, M. J., Nevin, N. C., Harris, R., Read, A. P., Fielding, D. W. and Walker, S. (1981). Vitamin supplementation and neural tube defects. *Lancet* **ii**, 1425.
140. Soltan, M. H. and Jenkins, D. M. (1982). Maternal and fetal plasma zinc concentration and fetal abnormality. *Brit. J. Obstet. Gynaecol.* **89**, 56–58.
141. Stein, Z., Susser, S., Warburton, D., Wittes, J. and Kline, J. (1975). Spontaneous abortion as a screening device: the effect of fetal survival on the incidence of birth defects. *Am. J. Epidemiol.* **102**, 275–290.
142. Stevenson, A. C., Johnston, H. A., Stewart, M. I. P. and Golding, D. R. (1966). Congenital Malformations: A Report of a Study of Series of Consecutive Births in 24 Centres. *Bull. WHO* **34**, *suppl.*
143. Thiersch, J. B. (1952). Therapeutic abortions with a folic acid antagonist, 4-aminopteroyl-glutamic acid (4-amino P.G.A.) administered by the oral route. *Am. J. Obstet. Gynecol.* **63**, 1298–1304.
144. Thiersch, J. B. (1956). The control of reproduction in rats with the aid of antimetabolites and early experiences with antimetabolites as abortifacient agents in man. *Acta Endocrinol.* **23**, Suppl. 28, 37–45.
145. Trimble, B. K. and Baird, P. A. (1978). Congenital anomalies of the central nervous system: Incidence in British Columbia, 1952–72. *Teratology* **17**, 43–49.
146. Tünte, W. (1964). Zur Häufigkeit der Anencephalie und Spina bifida aperta im Regierungsbezirk Münster. *Zeitschrift für Menschliche Vererbungs- und Konstitutionslehre* **37**, 525–530.
147. Tünte, W. (1968). Zur Frage der jahreszeitlichen Häufigkeit der Anencephalie. *Humangenetik* **6**, 225–236.
148. Verma, I. C. (1978). High frequency of neural-tube defects in north India. *Lancet* **i**, 879–880.
149. Verstege, J. C. W. (1971). "Anencephalie in Nederland 1951–1968." Centraal Bureau voor de Statistiek, Staatsuitgeverij, The Hague.
150. Warkany, J. (1947). Etiology of congenital malformations. *Adv. Pediatrics* **2**, 1–63.
151. WHO Scientific Group on Genetic Factors in Congenital Malformations (1970): Genetic factors in congenital malformations. *WHO Tech. Rep. Ser.* No. 438.
152. Williamson, E. M. (1965). Incidence and family aggregation of major congenital malformations of central nervous system. *J. Med. Genet.* **2**, 161–172.
153. Wilson, M. G. and Stein, A. M. (1969). Teratogenic effects of Asian influenza: an extended study. *J. Am. Med. Assoc.* **210**, 336–337.

154. Wilson, T. S. (1971). A study of congenital malformations of the central nervous system among Glasgow births 1964–1968. *Health Bull.* **29**, 79–87.
155. Wynne-Davies, R. (1975). Congenital vertebral anomalies: aetiology and relationship to spina bifida cystica. *J. Med. Genet.* **12**, 280–288.
156. Yen, S. and MacMahon, B. (1968). Genetics of anencephaly and spina bifida? *Lancet* **ii**, 623–626.

Commentary

Nicholas Wald: A number of points directly relevant to the vitamin hypothesis could be given in greater detail. For example:

(1) To what extent are the observational studies specific tests of the hypothesis? To what extent might confounding have arisen, and if it did, is it likely to have been sufficient to "explain" the effect?

(2) The recurrence risk and the general population risk of neural tube defect appears to vary by a factor of ten. Is it valid to suggest that this factor varies with the general population prevalence – is the difference statistically significant? If not, the data suggest that the occurrences and recurrences have the same causes and should therefore be amenable to the same intervention.

(3) Geographical variation in the birth prevalence of neural tube defects appears to be important, particularly if this can be related to geographical variations in vitamin intake. Does not this evidence argue against the vitamin hypothesis, since neural tube defects are rare in many regions where nutritional deficiency (including vitamin deficiencies) are common.

(4) The statement that antenatal diagnosis and termination of affected pregnancies seem to have accounted for only a small fraction of the changing birth prevalence of neural tube defects in England and Wales may be incorrect (see Figs 3 and 4, and paper by Bradshaw *et al.* (1)). There is no doubt that from about the mid-1970s there has been a sizable reduction in the birth prevalence of neural tube defects, but we do not know to what extent this represents a decline in incidence. The paper by Owen cited (ref. 116 in the paper by Leck), based on changes in birth prevalence over a selected short period of time in a selected relatively small area does not provide much separate evidence for a general decline in incidence. As with the national data, the decline started earlier and was greater for anencephaly than for spina bifida, suggesting that antenatal diagnosis and selective abortion may

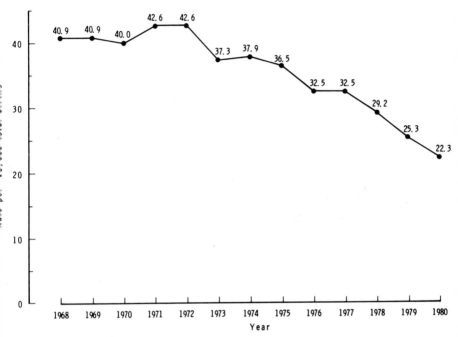

Fig. 3. Birth prevalence of central nervous system malformations in England and Wales. Source: OPCS.

have been an explanation for the decline. (The antenatal diagnosis of anencephaly by means of ultrasound was introduced before amniotic fluid or maternal serum alphafetoprotein testing.)

Figure 4 provides an indication of the extent of antenatal screening and selective abortion for open neural tube defects, but the data should be interpreted cautiously. CNS notifications (nearly all CNS notifications are neural tube defects) at birth are known to be incomplete, although there are data to indicate that no more than 10% or 20% of CNS malformations are unreported. The data relating to terminations of pregnancy are completely unvalidated. They are based upon statutory returns which medical practitioners complete and indicate in broad categories the reason for the termination, one of the categories being the risk of a fetal abnormality. Specifying the nature of the suspected abnormality is voluntary, so the number of notified terminations on account of a CNS abnormality must be incomplete. If more than 10–20% of such terminations are unre-

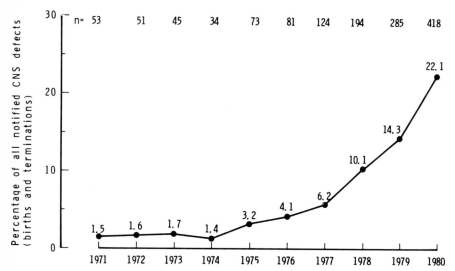

Fig. 4. Number (n) and percentage of central nervous system (CNS) malformations terminated in England and Wales. Source: OPCS.

ported, which is quite possible, Fig. 4 will underestimate the contribution which antenatal diagnosis and selective abortion is making to the declining birth prevalence of neural tube defects.

(5) The relationship between previous miscarriage and neural tube defects is important in the light of the fact that it appears to have confounded the results reported by Smithells and his colleagues (2, 3). Could the relationship be discussed in greater detail, and some quantitative estimates of the association be given?

(6) The last few pages of the paper are the most relevant and the most important, but they tend to be rather inconclusive. For example, the consistent results from many studies carry little weight if they share the same biases (p. 172). Is this a valid criticism? How does the vitamin hypothesis fit in with the various observations noted on pp. 172–173? Do the observations support or refute the hypothesis?

1. Bradshaw, J., Weale, J. and Weatherall, J. (1980). Congenital malformations of the central nervous system. *Population Trends* **19**, 13–18.
2. Smithells, R. W., Shepherd, S., Schorah, C. J., Seller, M. J., Nevin, N. C., Harris, R., Read, A. P. and Fielding, D. W. (1981). Apparent prevention of neural tube defects by vitamin supplementation. *Arch. Dis. Child.* **56**, 911–18.

3. Smithells, R. W., Schorah, C. J., Seller, M. J., Nevin, N. C., Harris, R., Read, A. P., Fielding, D. W., Walker, S. (1981). Vitamin supplementation and neural tube defects. *Lancet* ii, 1424–25.

Author's Reply: Data on the frequency of neural tube defects in England and Wales are presented in Figs 5–7. Figure 5 relates to spina bifida and shows national data on mortality (excluding stillbirths) for 1922–71 (6) and data for the city of Birmingham on mortality (including stillbirths) for 1940–53 and on birth prevalence for 1950–69 (2, 3). Both the national and the local figures peaked in 1942–3 and again in 1954–5. The main difference between the national and local figures is that the latter exceeded the former by an increasing margin. The excess is largely due to the Birmingham figures having included stillbirths and (from 1950 onwards) cases in children who survived infancy, the numbers in the latter category having increased substantially over the period covered by the Birmingham data. Figure 6 shows that the prevalence of anencephaly behaved like that of spina bifida, at least in Birmingham (2, 3).

Figure 7 relates to the prevalence since 1971 of all malformations of the central nervous system in England and Wales – here considered in preference to neural tube defects alone because the former but not the latter are among the indications for pregnancy termination for which data are given in the published legal abortion statistics (4). The most comprehensive national figures available for studying the birth prevalence of central nervous system defects are those obtained by combining data on stillbirths registered and liveborn children notified as having these defects (6). The lower line in Fig. 7

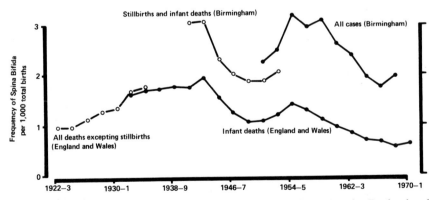

Fig. 5. Secular trends in indices of frequency of spina bifida: data for England and Wales on mortality (excluding stillbirths) (6) and Birmingham data on mortality (including stillbirths) (2) and prevalence at birth (3). The Birmingham statistics, but not those for England and Wales, include cases of encephalocoele.

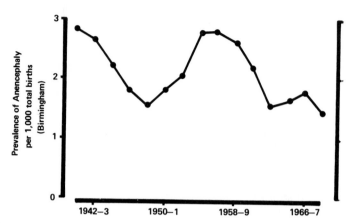

Fig. 6. Secular trend in prevalence at birth of anencephaly in Birmingham (2, 3).

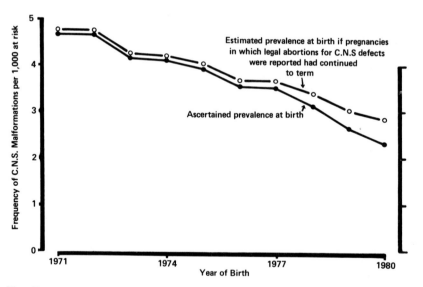

Fig. 7. Secular trends for England and Wales in (a) prevalence at birth of central nervous system defects that were reported on stillbirth certificates and on notifications of affected liveborn children (lower line) and (b) estimates of what the above prevalence would have been if the offspring of pregnancies in which legal abortion for fetal central nervous system defects was notified had also been born and reported to have defects (upper line).

shows that according to these data the prevalence of central nervous system defects fell by half between 1972 and 1980. The upper line shows estimates of what the prevalence would have been if the pregnancies in which legal abortion for fetal central nervous system defects was reported had continued to term, and if three-fifths of the resulting births had occurred in the same calendar year as the abortions and two-fifths in the next year. It was necessary to estimate the relevant abortion statistics for 1970 and 1978 from the data for adjacent years. The results suggest that the increase in the number of legal abortions carried out for defects of the central nervous system has only been sufficient to account for one-fifth of the decline in birth prevalence between 1972 and 1980.

Clearly this finding must be viewed with caution, since malformations of the newborn are not always notified, and the same may be true of abortions carried out for malformations of the central nervous system; but a local study in Liverpool in which more reliable methods were used gave very similar results (5). It would be interesting to compare the trend of birth prevalence over the last decade in England and Wales with that in the Irish Republic with its different policy on abortion. In one Dublin hospital series the prevalence of neural tube defects declined from 12 per 1000 in 1960–1 to 5 per 1000 in 1974–5 (1). The figure of 4·4 per 1000 given in Kirke's Table 1 for Dublin in 1980 is even lower, but one cannot tell whether to accept this as evidence of a further decline without knowing more about the populations on which the figures are based.

1. Elwood, J. M. and Elwood, J. H. (1980). "Epidemiology of Anencephalus and Spina Bifida." Oxford University Press, Oxford.
2. Leck, I. (1966). Changes in the incidence of neural tube defects. *Lancet* **ii**, 791–793.
3. Leck, I. (1981). Epidemiological aspects of paediatrics: insights into the causation of disorders of early life. *In* "Scientific Foundations of Paediatrics", 2nd edition (J. A. Davis and J. Dobbing, eds) pp. 947–979. Heinemann, London.
4. Office of Population Censuses and Surveys (1978–82). Abortion Statistics: Legal Abortions Carried Out under the Abortion Act in England and Wales, 1974–1980: Series AB, nos 1–7.
5. Owens, J. R., Harris, F., McAllister, E. and West, L. (1981). 19-year incidence of neural tube defects in area under constant surveillance. *Lancet* **ii**, 1032–1035.
6. Rogers, S. C. and Weatherall, J. A. C. (1976). "Anencephalus, Spina Bifida and Congenital Hydrocephalus: England and Wales, 1964–1972" (Studies on Medical and Population Studies No. 32). Her Majesty's Stationery Office, London.

Dick Smithells:

(1) The data on half-sibs and cousins indicate that maternal influences are more important than paternal observations consistent with a "maternal nutrition" hypothesis.

(2) Leck's observation that "trends in incidence brought about by aetiological influences are more likely than variations in miscarriage rates to be responsible for the association between the prevalence of NTD and at least some demographic factors" is also consistent with a "maternal nutrition" hypothesis. (However, as the nutritional hypothesis *derives from* epidemiological data, this is hardly surprising!)

(3) *The "trophoblastic rest" hypothesis.* I understand that trophoblastic tissue remaining *in utero* after miscarriage only lives as long as the pregnancy would have lasted (unless it becomes malignant). If this is true the hypothesis could be tested by looking at NTD incidence after miscarriage according to the time interval between miscarriage and next conception.

(4) "Folate deficiency seems at the present time more likely than any other nutritional problem . . .". Here I think Leck is making the same *potential* error as Laurence, namely, concentrating on folate because there is little information about other nutrients. If the nutritional mechanism is thought to be a *deficient diet* it is highly unlikely that a single nutrient is involved. It is almost impossible to devise a diet that is seriously deficient of folate but adequate for all other nutrients. The contribution of vitamin C cannot be studied in experimental animals because it is difficult to induce NTD in guinea pigs, and all other laboratory animals can synthesize vitamin C. If the nutritional mechanism is a *metabolic block*, folate is a strong candidate and the role of zinc fits in nicely, but if, as Laurence suggests, dietary counselling is effective, can there be a metabolic block?

In fairness to Leck, however, he recommends a high priority for studies of biochemistry other than folate, a proposal which has my enthusiastic support.

Felix Beck: Leck begins with a thoroughly admirable, in-depth study of the demographic variables associated to a greater or lesser degree with neural tube defects. As a result of this, one is left in no doubt of the strong genotypic influences underlying the failure of the neural tube to close. It is clearly shown that, although genotypic factors are of major importance, the form in which they manifest themselves is subject to speculation.

While the standard multifactorial model is clearly a strong candidate a number of factors are shown to cause its modification so that its predictive value is not great compared, for example, with that of the cleft palate model.

Leck then turns his attention to the zygote interaction model proposed by Knox which has been largely forgotten in the present discussion. The model has certain advantages which are mainly at present of a statistical nature and little exists in the way of positive proof for its biological identity. Recently, a paper by Huxham *et al.* (1) has produced some circumstantial evidence in its favour but in our present state of knowledge this cannot be regarded as being very strong.

Having made out the case that the standard multifactorial model may not be the only genotypic determinant underlying neural tube dysraphism, the author then proceeds to examine specific causes for neural tube defects. He reminds us of a number of theories previously in vogue and discounts those for which no positive scientific proof has been shown to exist. This leaves us with the undoubtedly raised level of neural tube defect in diabetes, its possible correlation with influenza and hyperthermia, its association with zinc deficiency and now (very strongly) its association with nutritional deficiencies, particularly certain vitamins including folate.

Leck's work is particularly apposite in reminding us of the relatively circumscribed nature of the present findings and of the continuing need to investigate other avenues in our quest to understand this important clinical condition.

1. Huxham, M., Gupta, M., Azoubel, R. and Beck, F. (1982). Dose Dependent Induction of Abnormalities *in vitro* by Tissue Homogenates of Placenta and Decidua. *Br. J. Exp. Path.* **63**, 95.

Michael Laurence: All epidemiological studies that depend on so-called "prevalence" figures have to be taken with caution as the true "incidence" of neual tube defects is almost certainly many times higher than the former. This is well illustrated by the figures in Leck's Table 1. It is almost certain that the many conceptuses which are lost in the first 8 weeks include an even greater proportion of NTD than the conceptuses that abort after 8 weeks. Nearly all epidemiological studies of NTD are therefore based on the small portion of the iceberg that projects out of the water. It is therefore dangerous to try and draw too firm conclusions on minutiae of epidemiological differences and variations. A small change in the early miscarriage rate could well produce major variations in the "prevalence" of recorded NTD especially if the change in the miscarriage rate differentially affects those fetuses with NTD.

NTD in a number of different communities seem to present as a quite distinct and separate problem. A large proportion of NTD in Britain consist of anencephaly and severe open spina bifida. In the north-west of the North American continent, anencephaly is rather less common than spina bifida, the widely open spina bifida is relatively uncommon and many of the latter are closed. In South-eastern Asia there is an equal proportion of males and females with spina bifida, and a relatively high proportion of them are encephalocoeles and anterior spina bifidas of the head, which are quite rare in Europe and North America. It is possible, or indeed probable that in these groups alone aetiological factors responsible for triggering off the malformations may be different from the factors operating in the British Isles and perhaps Europe.

As stated above the number of neural tube defects that miscarry are almost certainly a gross underestimate and therefore the "incidence" figures are a severe underestimate, especially as they refer to abortuses of 8 weeks or more (at least 40 days after conception) whereas the neural tube closure defect occurs 2–3 weeks earlier than that. Prenatal diagnosis of neural tube defects in high risk women is now fairly universal in England, Wales and Scotland. It is accepted that even the elimination of all recurrences would at most account for a 20% drop in the "prevalence" at or around term. However, in South Wales, a number of regions of England, and most of Scotland, maternal serum AFP screening is carried out on the majority of pregnancies and is in fact leading to the early antenatal detection of the majority of open neural tube defects and therefore to a considerable reduction in the "prevalence" of these at or around birth. In mid-Glamorgan where the incidence between 1956–62, and again 1964–6 was almost 8 per 1000 births, this had fallen to 4·7 per 1000 births by 1976–9 provided all the cases detected prenatally and terminated were included. Had these been excluded the "prevalence" would have been between 1 and 2 per 1000 births.

Spina bifida of the myelocoele and myelomeningocoele variety in South Wales, and for that matter also cases referred to the Hospital for Sick Children, Great Ormond Street (London) up to 1956 show the usual small preponderance of females. However, in females the condition seems to be either more severe or the complications are more severe for later in childhood the numbers of males to females become equal and by adolescence there is a preponderance of male survivors who also seem to be slightly less handicapped physically as well as mentally, than the surviving females.

Peadar Kirke: I have little to add to Leck's succinct and comprehensive review.

His estimate of the prevalence at birth of neural tube defects in England and Wales in 1980 (1·9 per 1000 total births) emphasizes the greater magnitude of this problem in Ireland. Data from the Eurocat Register of Congenital Malformations for 1980 confirm the relatively high prevalence at birth of neural tube defects in this country (Table 3) (3).

The prevalence at birth of neural tube defects has been falling throughout the United Kingdom in recent years (1, 5, 2). Elwood and Scott recently reported a substantial decline in the prevalence at birth of anencephalus in England and Wales, Northern Ireland and Scotland during the past decade (2). Perinatal mortality rates (late fetal plus first week deaths per 1000 total births) for anencephalus are shown in Fig. 8 for England and Wales, the Irish Republic, Northern Ireland and Scotland for the period 1966–79. The sources of data are the Office of Population Censuses and Surveys for England and Wales, the Central Statistics Office for the Irish Republic, the

Table 3. Prevalence at birth of neural tube defects per 1000 total births in selected Eurocat Registers in 1980. (3)

Register	Prevalence at birth	Total births
Dublin	4·38	26 245
Belfast	3·81	28 582
Glasgow	2·36	13 552
Liverpool	1·54	20 798

General Register Office for Northern Ireland and the General Register Office for Scotland. The secular trend in the Irish Republic was similar to those in Scotland and England and Wales until about 1973. The marked fall in mortality since 1975 in England and Wales, Northern Ireland and Scotland is not apparent in the Irish Republic although the trend there is also downward. The striking difference between the Irish Republic and the rest of the British Isles in secular trends in anencephalus since the early 1970's is illustrated in Table 4. There is no obvious explanation for the different experience of the Irish Republic. Antenatal diagnosis and termination of affected pregnancies is not practised in the Irish Republic but there is general agreement that therapeutic abortion accounts for only a small fraction of the decline in neural tube defects in the United Kingdom countries (5, 2, 4).

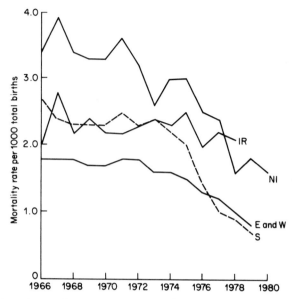

Fig. 8. Perinatal mortality rates for anencephalus in England and Wales (E and W), the Irish Republic (IR), Northern Ireland (NI) and Scotland (S) 1966–79.

1. Bradshaw, J., Weale, J. and Weatherall, J. (1980). Congenital malformations of the central nervous system. *Population Trends* **19**, 13–8.
2. Elwood, J. H. (1982). Scott, M. J. Prevalence of anencephalus in the United Kingdom. *Devel. Med. Child Neurol.* **24**, 394–5.
3. Eurocat, Central Register (1982). Registration of Congenital Abnormalities and Multiple Births. Third Report 1980. Eurocat Central Register. Brussels.
4. Leck, I. (1983). This volume, pp. 155–174.
5. Nevin, N. C. (1981). Neural tube defects. *Lancet* **ii**, 1290–1.

Norman Nevin: This paper is a thorough and comprehensive review of the epidemiology of neural tube defects (NTDs), emphasizing that their frequency is dependent on two groups of variables, namely, demographic and environmental factors. Most at the Workshop will agree with his statement that there is a "dearth of good evidence incriminating specific teratogens". The field of neural tube defects is littered with the wrecks of hypotheses which have failed to stand the rigors of time. This paper succintly reviews the current thinking concerning the aetiological factors involved in the causation of NTDs.

I have the following comments:

(1) There is no mention of whether iniencephaly is included with NTDs in the definition of neural tube defects.

Table 4. Average perinatal mortality rates (per 1000 total births) for anencephalus in 1970–1 and 1977–8 in England and Wales, the Irish Republic, Northern Ireland and Scotland.

	Perinatal mortality rates 1970–71	1977–78	% fall
England and Wales	1·8	1·1	38·9
Irish Republic	2·2	2·1	4·5
Northern Ireland	3·5	2·0	42·9
Scotland	2·4	1·0	58·3

(2) "Prevalence" and "incidence". There has been confusion in the use of these terms. Traditionally, the occurrence of malformations has been described in terms of incidence per 1000 births. Naggan (3) suggested that it is more appropriate to consider the rates of occurrence of NTDs as point prevalence rates, that is the prevalence at birth. "Prevalence" is thus defined as the frequency of a disease or a disorder at a designated point in time. Little knowledge exists as to the true "incidence" of the NTDs because of early fetal loss. Others (6, 7) share Leck's use of "prevalence" and "incidence".

(3) Leck highlights some of the difficulties in estimating even the prevalence at birth. Despite the lethality of many NTDs, not all will be reported on the official birth documents. Our experience has been similar (5). In Northern Ireland for three years (1974–6), using multiple sources of ascertainment, a total of 686 infants with NTDs was identified among 79 783 live and stillbirths. The official sources of ascertainment, the Registrar General's Congenital Malformation Notification System, and the Child Health System, however, together only identified 86·2% of all these NTDs.

(4) Leck makes a good point that the incidence of NTDs (from studies of abortions) can only be regarded as very tentative. Evidence is accumulating on the heterogeneity of NTDs (1, 2) and different aetiologic factors may be involved from conception to birth.

(5) In the United Kingdom, many areas within the past decade, have experienced a decline in the prevalence at birth of NTDs. It is probably correct that "antenatal diagnosis and termination of affected pregnancies seems to have accounted for only a small fraction of this decline". For the period 1974 to 1979 in Northern Ireland, the prevalence of NTDs at birth was 6·0 per 1000 total births, and when pregnancies terminated because of an NTD were included, the prevalence rose only to 6·25 per 1000. It was clear that prenatal diagnosis

and termination could not account for the observed decrease in birth prevalence (4).

(6) The term "rachischisis" should be avoided.

(7) Although favouring folic acid as probably the effective constituent in the prevention of NTDs, Leck is correct when he recommends a high priority for studies of biochemistry other than folate.

1. Holmes, L. B., Driscoll, S. G. and Atkins, L. A. (1976). Etiologic heterogeneity of neural tube defects. *New Eng. J. Med.* **294**, 365–369.
2. Khoury, M. J., Erickson, J. D. and James, L. M. (1982). Etiologic heterogeneity of neural tube defects: clues from epidemiology. *Am. J. Epidemiol.* **115**, 538–548.
3. Naggan, L. (1976). I. Methodology of ascertainment in international comparisons. II Anencephaly and spina bifida in Israel. *In* "Birth Defects: Risks and Consequences" (S. Kelly, E. B. Hook, D. T. Janerich and I. H. Porter, eds) pp. 41–58. Academic Press, New York and London.
4. Nevin, N. C. (1981). Neural tube defects. *Lancet* **ii**, 1290–1291.
5. Nevin, N. C., McDonald, J. R. and Walby, A. L. (1978). A comparison of neural tube defects identified by two independent routine recording systems for congenital malformations in Northern Ireland. *Int. J. Epidemiol.* **7**, 319–321.
6. Sever, L. E. (1978). Epidemiologic aspects of neural tube defects *In* "The Prevention of Neural Tube Defects: The Role of Apha-fetoprotein" (B. R. Crandall and M. A. B. Brazier, eds) pp. 75–89. Academic Press, New York.
7. Sever, L. E., Sanders, M. and Monsen, R. (1982). An epidemiologic study of neural tube defects in Los Angeles County. 1. Prevalence at birth based on multiple sources of ascertainment. *Teratology* **25**, 315–321.

John Edwards: The distinction of related and causal seems valuable; it seems logical to put the secondary effects second. Sometimes the primary and secondary nature cannot be asserted. An example is the crucial problem of reduced birth weights in neural tube defects.

The confusion due to using spina bifida as a synonym of craniorrhachischisis is unfortunate, even if fairly harmless. The conditions are distinct, and myelocoele is rarely seen with anencephaly. The term "prevalence" is now difficult unless "birth" includes termination.

The "standard multifactorial model" merely means relatives are similar and insults have an additive effect on injury. I do not think the term "standard multifactorial model" useful, as it implies that predictions can be made with numbers better than with words. If it must have a name, then the "Hippocratic model" would be correct, or possibly Pare's model, who was specific on malformations. It's mathematical description was explicit in Karl Pearson's work of around 1904 in many examples justifying his tetrachoric coefficients (see early issues of *Biometrica*). The use of the term "multifactorial" has been a major obstacle to the search for a major, or "unifactorial" aggravating factor. The word could usefully be excluded from scientific medicine. As Leck says "It seems blatantly obvious that aetiological influences must include both the genotype and other factors".

Heritability can only be calculated if there are no familial environmental features. The use of this word in man, especially in relation to events strongly associated with environmental features, is confusing. If it is used, it is important to appreciate that "heritability" and "opportunity for effective environmental action" are formally irrelevant. An obvious example is starvation, which, in practice, is highly familial in deprived areas. Knox's model is necessarily additive to a general familial tendency, and there is no reason to suppose that obvious consequences of relations being similar should be regarded as opposing Knox's model in which spouses are sufficiently different to produce relevant immunological responses. The strongest evidence against Knox's model as sufficient to account for more than a minority is the variability in space and time and the higher incidence in first births.

Chris Schorer: I have few comments to make on Leck's thorough review of epidemiological aspects of the causation of neural tube defects but have devoted more space to a consideration of the appendix. One observation in the main paper is of particular interest. Leck reports that apart from dietary factors the only other environmental influences that appear to be associated with an excess of NTD malformations are diabetes and hyperthermia. It is of relevance that we have recently found low blood folic acid concentrations in a number of diabetics. (Percent of diabetics with folate less than lower limit of normal: red cell 35%; serum 25%) and there has also been a report indicating altered folate metabolism in subjects with hyperthermia (1).

1. Osifo, B. O. A., Lukanmbi, F. A. and Familusi, J. B. (1981). Increase of body temperature and folic acid metabolism. *Acta Vitaminol. Enzymol.* 3 N.S., 177.

Appendix I

Maternal diet and nutrition during early pregnancy and after delivery in North London

IAN LECK, C. A. ILES, I. M. SHARMAN, THANE TOE
AND G. R. WADSWORTH

Department of Community Medicine, University of Manchester;
Medical Unit, University College Hospital Medical School, London;
Dunn Nutritional Laboratory, University of Cambridge and
Medical Research Council; and Department of Human Nutrition,
London School of Hygiene and Tropical Medicine.

Summary

The feasibility of using data on diet in early pregnancy and on diet and blood chemistry after delivery to identify women whose blood levels of nutrients may have been abnormal during early pregnancy was explored in 168 patients of a London obstetric unit. Particular attention was paid to vitamin A and folate.

Erythrocyte levels of folate and serum levels of folate, vitamin A and carotenoids in early pregnancy were only weakly correlated with dietary intake of the corresponding vitamins at the same time or a year later, but correlations between the levels of erythrocyte folate and serum carotenoids in early pregnancy and the corresponding levels a year later were higher.

Blood folate levels tended to be relatively low in mothers of malformed children, and also in the social classes and months in which the risks of developing neural tube defects seem to be especially high.

It is concluded that biochemical comparisons between women who have fairly recently borne malformed and normal children might help to clarify the relationship of nutrition to teratogenesis.

Introduction

One message of the present workshop must surely be that even if and when it is confirmed that human neural tube defects can be prevented by nutritional measures, further studies of diet and nutrition in the mothers of malformed and normal children will be needed to explain these findings. Insofar as the nutrients taken by the mother influence embryonic development, they presumably do so by affecting the quantities in which they or their derivatives are available to the conceptus. As these quantities are likely to be related more closely to the levels of nutrients in the mother's body than to the levels in her diet, particular attention needs to be paid to the analysis of blood and other tissues, and to assessing the relative importance of dietary and constitutional factors in determining tissue levels.

An ideal way to explore these issues might be to collect dietary data and tissue samples within about a month of conception, and then to compare the nutritional data for pregnancies in which the offspring was subsequently found to be malformed with data for the other pregnancies; but it would be immensely difficult if not impossible to collect such data from the thousands of women that would be needed to obtain an adequate number of malformed children. A much less demanding approach, which would seem to be acceptable if women's diets and tissue levels of nutrients were sufficiently stable, would be to measure and compare these variables in women who had previously had a malformed child and in matched controls.

The research described in this Appendix had two main objectives. The first was to determine whether dietary and blood levels of certain nutrients (mainly folate and vitamin A) remain stable enough between early pregnancy and a year later to justify retrospective comparisons of those variables in the mothers of malformed and normal children. The second objective was to assess how closely the blood levels of these nutrients are correlated with dietary as opposed to constitutional factors. The decision to focus particularly on the situation one year after early pregnancy was made in order that whatever similarity there was between the findings during and after pregnancy might not be weakened by seasonal variations. Of the two vitamins given especial attention, folate was chosen because of some of the evidence reviewed in the above paper, and vitamin A because of the capacity of hypervitaminosis A to produce neural tube defects in other mammals (which Seller's paper (pp. 1–14) documents) and the reports that high vitamin A levels are commoner than average in the livers of infants with neural tube defects and in serum from mothers of such infants (3, 7).

Data Collection

The subjects for the research were women of British or Irish origin who attended the antenatal booking clinic of the professorial obstetric unit at University College Hospital, London, within 12 weeks of the onset of their last menses, during a 12-month period in 1968–9. They were recruited by an experienced research dietitian (CAI), who attended each clinic, arranged for venous blood samples to be taken there from the women who agreed to participate, and made a home visit a day or two later to each of these women.

The main purpose of this home visit was to arrange for the woman to keep a dietary diary for 7 consecutive days, including so far as possible the weight of each item (obtained by cumulative weighing when more than one item was served on the same plate). To this end she was provided with a flat-topped spring balance and a diet record book like those described by Topp *et al.* (16), together with printed and verbal instructions. During and at the end of the week for which the diary was kept, each woman was normally visited three more times by the dietitian, who made her own assessment of the reliability of the woman's diary and also completed a questionnaire about dietary habits, socioeconomic circumstances, reproductive and family history, and general health.

During the period when these women were due to be delivered, the dietitian regularly visited the relevant obstetric wards and arranged in most cases for further venous blood samples to be taken during the puerperium.

Finally, the dietitian tried to get in touch with each woman again one year after recruiting her to the study. It was then arranged that those who were willing to collaborate again should keep a dietary diary for a second seven-day period, using the same procedures as before. At the same time, most of these women provided further venous blood samples, which were collected by a medically qualified research worker (TT) who accompanied the dietitian on some of her visits.

When first seen at the antenatal clinic, 168 women agreed to participate. Blood samples were obtained from all 168 women at this time, from 139 during the puerperium, and from 103 12 months after entry, although it was not possible to measure the level of each substance of interest in every one of these cases. Seven-day dietary diaries were completed by 142 of the 168 women at the time they entered the study, and by 108 a year later. Given the community served by the antenatal clinic and the exclusion of women who booked more than 12 weeks after their last menses, it was inevitable that primigravidae and women of high socioeconomic status would be over-represented in the study, the latter grossly so; but these biases do not invalidate the use of the data to compare diet with blood picture, or prenatal findings with post-natal, within the same individuals.

Methods of Analysis

Each item of food in the dietary diaries was coded by the dietitian. A computer programme written in the Department of Clinical Epidemiology and Social Medicine, St. Thomas's Hospital Medical School, and described by Topp *et al.* (16), was then used to convert the dietary data into estimates of each woman's mean daily intake of energy and of the principal nutrients and foods during each of the weeks surveyed. All the food codes and conversion tables used had been produced in 1969 by the Department of Health and Social Security of the United Kingdom, with one exception: these tables did not cover folate content, for which the figures for *Lactobacillus casei* active folates ("free folate") in common foods given by Hurdle (5, 6) were used.

Each blood sample was divided initially into two portions, one being mixed with sequestrin and the other allowed to clot. Blood from the first of these portions was used (a) for haemoglobin estimation by the cyanmethae-moglobin method as modified by van Kampen and Zilstra (2); (b) for estimating the packed cell volume by micro-haematocrit; and (c) for assay-ing whole blood folate activity by the microbiological method with *L. casei* that Hoffbrand (4) describes. Serum from the other portion of blood was used (a) to assay serum folate activity, again with *L. casei*, by the method of Waters and Mollin (18); (b) to measure total serum proteins by the Biuret method as described by Wootton (19); and (c) to estimate serum levels of carotenoids and retinol by a colorimetric method in which carotenoids are measured by their natural yellow colour and retinol by the blue colour produced by the antimony trichloride reagent (10). All these analyses were done in the Department of Human Nutrition, London School of Hygiene and Tropical Medicine, except for the carotenoid and retinol determina-tions, which were carried out in the Dunn Nutritional Laboratory. Erythro-cyte folate activity e for each blood sample was estimated from activity in whole blood b and in serum s and from the packed cell volume (corrected for trapped plasma) per unit blood volume p, using the formula:

$$e = \frac{b - s(1 - p)}{p}$$

To obtain p, observed packed cell volume (p') was multiplied by ($0 \cdot 99161 - 0 \cdot 0352p'$) – the factor implied by Wadsworth's formula for estimating the volume of trapped plasma (17).

Results

Dietary Intakes

Dietary diaries for two weeks, one in early pregnancy and one a year later, were completed by 106 women, and the estimates of mean daily intake of energy, energy sources, vitamin A and folate yielded by their diaries for these two weeks are compared in the left half of Table 1. Vitamin A and folate obtained from tablets prescribed at the antenatal clinic have been excluded from the first week estimates, since they would not have been taken soon enough to influence either embryonic development or the vitamin levels in the initial blood samples. For each nutrient the mean intake for the study population was higher in early pregnancy than a year later, and the product-moment coefficients of correlation between first and second week means for individuals were between $0 \cdot 32$ and $0 \cdot 54$.

Before these coefficients are accepted as indices of the extent to which diet after delivery reflects the situation at the time when the embryo is developing, the possibility of bias by inaccurate record-keeping must be considered: if for example there were women who habitually kept incomplete diaries, both in the first week and in the second, this would tend to inflate the coefficients. Separate analyses were therefore carried out on the data relating to the women judged by the dietitian to have kept diaries of particularly high quality. There were 55 of these "good recorders", including 43 who had completed diaries for both weeks. Data for these 43 women are given in the right half of Table 1. As one would expect, the recorded intake of each nutrient was higher for them than for all women, and this was particularly true for vitamin A and folate. The "good recorders' " first and second week intakes of these vitamins were more highly correlated than those of all women, but the reverse was true for the energy sources.

It was thought that higher correlations might be achieved by excluding one or more of four groups of mothers who might have had particular reason to modify their diets, perhaps as part of a more general change in life-style, between the first and second weeks. The four groups in question were those suffering from nausea or vomiting of pregnancy during the first week, those

Table 1. Diet recorded in early pregnancy and one year later.

Nutrient	All subjects ($n = 106$) Mean daily intake ± s.d. of means for individuals Early pregnancy	One year later	Correlation coefficient	"Good recorders" ($n = 43$) Mean daily intake ± s.d. of means for individuals Early pregnancy	One year later	Correlation coefficient
Calories	2196 ± 412	2005 ± 466	0·44	2371 ± 410	2260 ± 418	0·28
Protein (g)	77 ± 17	73 ± 18	0·54	84 ± 15	82 ± 18	0·35
Fat (g)	102 ± 23	95 ± 26	0·48	110 ± 22	107 ± 24	0·42
Carbohydrate (g)	249 ± 60	212 ± 62	0·46	262 ± 60	236 ± 52	0·32
Vitamin A (μg retinol equivalent)	1313 ± 1058[a]	1245 ± 857	0·32	1593 ± 1210[a]	1493 ± 844	0·51
Free folate (μg)	187 ± 99[a]	154 ± 78	0·49	221 ± 110[a]	193 ± 88	0·56

[a] Figures exclude vitamin tablets.

breast-feeding during the second, those doing paid work on a more than half-time basis at either time, and those who had no surviving children apart from the one born during the study. The correlation coefficients for the "good recorders" were therefore recomputed after excluding each of these four categories in turn, but none of the resulting sets of figures (Table 2) was consistently higher than those for all "good recorders".

Although not a primary concern of this study, the relationship of diet and nutrition in early pregnancy to socioeconomic status and season merits some attention in view of the seasonal and social class trends in the prevalence of neural tube defects. Of the 142 women who completed a dietary diary in early pregnancy, 137 could be classified by husband's social class according to the Registrar-General's *Classification of Occupations* (11). Mean daily intakes in early pregnancy for those with husbands in social classes I and II (professional and managerial occupations) and for the remainder of the 137 are compared in the left half of Table 3. At first sight, these figures appear to suggest that the women of social classes I and II had the higher intake of energy and of each nutrient with the exception of carbohydrates. However, these differences seem in large part to be due to the prevalence of "good recorders" in social classes I and II (53%) being higher than in the other classes (23%): among the "good recorders" in the two social groups (compared in the right half of Table 3), the difference in calorie intake was reversed and only the vitamin A and folate levels remained substantially higher in social classes I and II.

The range of seasonal variation in diet in early pregnancy (Table 4) also seemed to be greater for the vitamins examined than for the energy sources. The seasons of high intake were April–June for vitamin A and January–June for free folate, and in each of these cases the difference between the high-intake season and the rest of the year was more than twice its standard error. However, the trends shown would only be accurate if there was no seasonal variation in the vitamin content of individual foods, since the food conversion tables that were used do not allow for any such variation.

Blood Levels

The haematological studies in early pregnancy and the puerperium yielded the results shown in Table 5 for the women whose blood was sampled on both occasions. Between these times many of the women were on vitamin supplements, and increases occurred in all the means for the vitamins and vitamin precursor measured. The two measures of folate showed a greater relative increase than the two related to vitamin A; and within each of these pairs, there was a greater increase in the variable that reflects more closely the vitamin's availability within the body over a long period (erythrocyte

Table 2. Correlation coefficients between diet recorded in early pregnancy and one year later by various subgroups of "good recorders".

			Correlation coefficients		
Nutrient	All "good recorders" (n = 43)	"Good recorders" with no nausea/vomiting in first study week (n = 24)	"Good recorders" not breast-feeding in second study week (n = 31)	"Good recorders" with no paid work[b] in either study week (n = 20)	"Good recorders" with surviving elder child(ren) (n = 12)
Calories	0·28	0·45	0·25	−0·18	0·27
Protein	0·35	0·34	0·29	−0·04	0·01
Fat	0·42	0·54	0·42	0·19	0·41
Carbohydrate	0·32	0·50	0·41	0·22	0·52
Vitamin A[a]	0·51	0·41	0·68	0·52	0·23
Free folate[a]	0·56	0·48	0·54	0·42	0·56

[a] Not including vitamin tablets in early pregnancy. [b] Including mothers doing paid work for less than 20 hours/week.

Table 3. Mean daily intake of certain nutrients recorded in early pregnancy, by social class of husband.

Nutrient	All subjects of defined social class		"Good recorders" of defined social class	
	Social classes I and II $(n = 77)$	Social classes III–V $(n = 60)$	Social classes I and II $(n = 41)$	Social classes III–V $(n = 14)$
Calories	2226	2090	2333	2385
Protein (g)	80	70	84	81
Fat (g)	105	96	110	108
Carbohydrate (g)	244	248	252	283
Vitamin A (μg retinol equivalent)[a]	1560	1060	1787	1455
Free folate (μg)[a]	213	151	230	181

[a] Figures exclude vitamin tablets.

Table 4. Mean daily intake of certain nutrients recorded in early pregnancy, by season.

Nutrient	Jan–March (n = 28)	April–June (n = 36)	July–Sept (n = 43)	Oct–Dec (n = 35)
Calories	2213	2157	2153	2128
Protein (g)	81	75	75	72
Fat (g)	104	99	100	99
Carbohydrate (g)	243	250	244	245
Vitamin A (μg retinol equivalent)[a]	1344	1664[b]	1095	1233
Free folate (μg)[a]	207	203	170	168

[a] Figures exclude vitamin tablets. [b] Difference from mean for remainder of year exceeds twice the standard error of this difference (computed using the standard deviation for all mothers in Table 10).

folate, serum retinol) than in the one more sensitive to short-term variations in intake (serum folate, serum carotenoids). The coefficient of correlation between individual levels in early pregnancy and the puerperium was above half for serum carotenoids, but the levels of other substances measured were much less closely correlated.

In the blood samples that were obtained one year after making the initial observations (Table 6), the mean for serum retinol showed a further increase, but those for folate and serum carotenoids were lower than the puerperal values and closer to the initial means. The correlations between the values observed initially and a year later were broadly comparable to those between the initial and puerperal values, with one exception: for erythrocyte folate the coefficient was less than one eighth between the initial and puerperal levels and more than a half between the initial levels and those of a year later.

During early pregnancy, all the mean blood vitamin levels studied were lower in the women with husbands in social classes III–V than in those of social classes I and II (Table 7), and the differences for serum carotenoids

Table 5. Blood levels in early pregnancy and puerperium.

Blood constituent	n	Mean ± s.d. Early pregnancy	Puerperium	Correlation coefficient
Haemoglobin (g%)	134	13·7 ± 1·1	13·5 ± 1·5	0·34
Serum proteins (g%)	133	7·4 ± 0·4	7·1 ± 0·5	0·13
Serum retinol (μg/ml)	125	0·33 ± 0·09	0·40 ± 0·12	0·00
Serum carotenoids (μg/ml)	125	1·15 ± 0·52	1·24 ± 0·45	0·58
Erythrocyte folate (ng/ml)	122	316 ± 115	514 ± 282	0·12
Serum folate (ng/ml)	130	9·7 ± 4·8	12·1 ± 8·1	0·28

Table 6. Blood levels in early pregnancy and one year later.

Blood constituent	n	Mean ± s.d. Early pregnancy	One year later	Correlation coefficient
Haemoglobin (g%)	102	13·7 ± 1·0	14·1 ± 1·0	0·26
Serum proteins (g%)	102	7·4 ± 0·4	7·7 ± 0·4	0·25
Serum retinol (μg/ml)	91	0·32 ± 0·09	0·44 ± 0·14	0·08
Serum carotenoids (μg/ml)	91	1·12 ± 0·49	1·11 ± 0·51	0·53
Erythrocyte folate (ng/ml)	98	303 ± 107	304 ± 151	0·53
Serum folate (ng/ml)	102	9·4 ± 4·5	10·3 ± 6·4	0·34

and serum and erythrocyte folate were all highly significant ($t \geqslant 3$). The trend with season (Table 8) was more variable, the quarters with the lowest means being October–December for serum carotenoids, January–March for serum retinol, and April–June for erythrocyte and serum folate. Only for two of these variables, serum carotenoids and erythrocyte folate, was the difference between the quarter with the lowest mean and the rest of the year greater than twice its standard error; but this criterion of significance was also satisfied by seasonal peaks which the means for serum folate and for haemoglobin reached in July–September.

Correlations between diet and blood levels

For each of the four blood vitamin levels examined, four coefficients of correlation with the dietary intake of the corresponding vitamin were computed, two for all available subjects and two for the "good recorders" among them (Table 9). The first coefficient of each pair relates blood level in early pregnancy to diet at about the same time, and was computed mainly in the hope of clarifying how much of the variance of tissue vitamin levels during

Table 7. Mean blood levels in early pregnancy, by social class of husband.

Blood constituent	Social classes I and II ($n \geqslant 81$)	Social classes III–V ($n \geqslant 71$)
Haemoglobin (g%)	13·6	13·7
Serum proteins (g%)	7·4	7·4
Serum retinol (μg/ml)	0·34	0·31
Serum carotenoids (μg/ml)[a]	1·29	0·98
Erythrocyte folate (ng/ml)[a]	344	288
Serum folate (ng/ml)[a]	11·0	8·5

[a] Difference between means exceeds twice its standard error (computed by using the standard deviation for all mothers in Table 10).

Table 8. Mean blood levels in early pregnancy, by season.

Blood constituent	Jan–March ($n \geqslant 34$)	April–June ($n \geqslant 40$)	July–Sept ($n \geqslant 46$)	Oct–Dec ($n \geqslant 38$)
Haemoglobin (g%)	13·4	13·7	14·1[a]	13·4
Serum proteins (g%)	7·4	7·5	7·5	7·4
Serum retinol (μg/ml)	0·30	0·34	0·34	0·32
Serum carotenoids (μg/ml)	1·25	1·18	1·19	0·94[a]
Erythrocyte folate (ng/ml)	360	268[a]	301	354
Serum folate (ng/ml)	10·3	8·7	11·3[a]	8·8

[a] Difference from mean for remainder of year exceeds twice the standard error of this difference (computed using the standard deviation for all mothers in Table 10).

pregnancy is dietary. The other coefficient of each pair relates blood level in early pregnancy to diet a year later, with a view to assessing whether any valid evidence as to the levels of vitamins available to developing embryos is likely to be obtained by observing their mothers' diets after the resulting infants have been born and examined.

The coefficients of correlation between blood levels in early pregnancy and diet at the same time all lay between 0·19 and 0·29, except that serum retinol and dietary vitamin A were less closely related. Each blood level was correlated almost as closely with intake a year later as with intake at the same time, except that erythrocyte folate showed no relationship to dietary folate a year later. The coefficients for the "good recorders" were similar to those for all subjects.

Mothers of malformed children

The need for more rigorous studies of the nutrition of women with malformed children, especially in early pregnancy, and the lack of data on which to base such studies, has created a case for publishing even very small bodies of data of this kind, in order to facilitate the pooling of such data from different sources and to provide leads for more extensive studies in the future. Two of the study pregnancies in the present series yielded children with malformations of embryonic origin (one cleft lip, and one Pierre Robin anomalad including cleft palate), and in two which yielded normal children there was a history of an elder sib with such a defect (one anencephaly – in a twin – and one spina bifida). Dietary and haematological data for the mothers of these four children are tabulated in Table 10. The most striking feature of these data is the blood folate levels. In three mothers of the four, the serum folate level was more than one standard deviation below the mean when first measured and again on one subsequent occasion. The same was true of the erythrocyte folate levels for two of these three mothers, including

Table 9. Correlation between dietary and blood levels of vitamins.

Variables correlated	All subjects				"Good recorders"			
	n	Mean blood level per ml	Mean daily intake	Correlation coefficient	n	Mean blood level per ml	Mean daily intake	Correlation coefficient
Serum retinol, vitamin A intake								
Levels in early pregnancy	137	0·33 µg	1340 µg[a]	0·09	54	0·35 µg	1718 µg[a]	0·02
Blood level in early pregnancy, intake one year later	103	0·33 µg	1252 µg	0·08	41	0·33 µg	1513 µg	0·05
Serum carotenoids, vitamin A intake								
Levels in early pregnancy	137	1·15 µg	1340 µg[a]	0·29	54	1·26 µg	1718 µg[a]	0·21
Blood level in early pregnancy, intake one year later	103	1·13 µg	1252 µg	0·26	41	1·21 µg	1513 µg	0·27
Erythrocyte folate, free folate intake								
Levels in early pregnancy	139	317 ng	185 µg[a]	0·23	55	351 ng	216 µg[a]	0·20
Blood level in early pregnancy, intake one year later	106	309 ng	152 µg	0·00	42	334 ng	190 µg	−0·07
Serum folate, free folate intake								
Levels in early pregnancy	141	9·7 ng	184 µg[a]	0·28	55	10·4 ng	216 µg[a]	0·19
Blood level in early pregnancy, intake one year later	107	9·4 ng	151 µg	0·27	42	9·7 ng	190 µg	0·32

[a] Figures exclude vitamin supplements.

Table 10. Dietary and blood levels in mothers of children with malformations of embryonic origin and in all mothers.

Details of case	Case no. 49 Child of index pregnancy had Pierre Robin anomalad (including cleft palate)	Case no. 124 Child of index pregnancy had cleft lip	Case no. 78 Child of previous pregnancy (twin) had anencephaly	Case no. 143 Child of previous pregnancy had spina bifida	Whole series (mean ± s.d.)
Daily intake					
Calories					
Initial	2642[b]	2003	2081	—	2160 ± 425
Final	2055	2191	2010	—	1982 ± 490
Protein (g)					
Initial	86	82	72	—	75 ± 17
Final	74	71	62	—	73 ± 19
Fat (g)					
Initial	101	92	85	—	100 ± 23
Final	106	100	80	—	94 ± 27
Carbohydrate (g)					
Initial	368[c]	224	263	—	246 ± 60
Final	211	265	275[b]	—	209 ± 64
Vitamin A (μg)					
Initial[a]	657	816	858	—	1322 ± 1024
Final	777	1140	744	—	1228 ± 858
Free folate (μg)					
Initial[a]	143	157	169	—	185 ± 94
Final	107	117	144	—	152 ± 78

Blood levels

Haemoglobin (g%)					
Initial	13·2	15·2[b]	13·7	14·8	13·7 ± 1·1
Puerperal	14·6	16·4[b]	12·5	12·8	13·6 ± 1·5
Final	15·6[b]	15·2[b]	13·5	–	14·1 ± 1·0
Serum proteins (g%)					
Initial	7·5	7·4	7·3	7·5	7·4 ± 0·4
Puerperal	7·0	7·3	–	6·7	7·1 ± 0·5
Final	7·9	8·0	7·5	–	7·7 ± 0·4
Serum retinol (μg/ml)					
Initial	0·32	0·30	0·36	0·28	0·33 ± 0·09
Puerperal	0·49	0·26[d]	–	0·29	0·40 ± 0·12
Final	0·55	0·46	0·25[d]	–	0·44 ± 0·14
Serum carotenoids (μg/ml)					
Initial	1·37	0·50[d]	0·79	0·84	1·14 ± 0·51
Puerperal	1·03	0·92	–	1·07	1·22 ± 0·45
Final	0·99	0·34[d]	0·53[d]	–	1·10 ± 0·51
Erythrocyte folate (ng/ml)					
Initial	141[d]	334	37[c]	306	318 ± 115
Puerperal	509	664	–	314	515 ± 281
Final	143[d]	238	17[d]	–	302 ± 149
Serum folate (ng/ml)					
Initial	3·4[d]	7·6	1·2[d]	4·2[d]	9·8 ± 5·1
Puerperal	18·0	21·4	–	2·0[d]	12·2 ± 8·1
Final	3·2[d]	7·0	1·8[d]	–	10·0 ± 6·3

[a] Figures exclude vitamin supplements. [b] Value > 1 s.d. above mean. [c] Value > 2 s.d. above mean. [d] Value > 1 s.d. below mean. [e] Value > 2 s.d. below mean.

Ian Leck et al.

one (the mother of the anencephalic) whose erythrocyte folate levels in early pregnancy and a year later were both less than half as high as those of any other mother in the study, although her estimated free folate intake was close to the mean each time. In the one mother with unremarkable folate levels who had a malformed child, the only findings that seem to invite comment are a consistently high haemoglobin concentration, and two serum carotenoid levels of more than one standard deviation below the mean.

Discussion

At the present time we have few if any more direct ways of measuring the amounts of vitamins and other nutrients available to the developing human embryo than to measure the levels of these nutrients in the mother's blood. Evidence that some such levels are correlated with the risk of malformations already exists in Smithells' report of low first-trimester blood vitamin levels – notably of erythrocyte folate – in pregnancies where the offspring had malformations of the central nervous system and (to a lesser degree) in the three social classes (III–V) where neural tube defects are commoner than average (14). Comparable evidence of a connection between low blood folate levels and malformations is provided by several of our own findings: the repeatedly low individual levels observed in three of the four women who had children with malformations of embryonic origin either in the index pregnancies or previously (Table 10), and the relatively low mean levels in early pregnancy observed not only in social classes III–V (Table 7) but also during the second quarter of the year – the quarter when offspring due to be born in winter (among whom the prevalence of neural tube defects at birth reaches its seasonal peak) pass through embryonic life (Table 8).

These findings give added relevance to the present study's main aim, which was to explore what evidence about the blood levels of nutrients in early pregnancy can be gleaned from information about either the diet at the same time or the diet or blood a year later. Whilst an ideal study of this issue would perhaps use haematological observations from 3 to 4 weeks after conception, rather than the later observations (largely from 8 to 10 weeks) which we used, the latter data may be as good a substitute for the former as can readily be obtained.

Our analysis of the relationship that diet bears to blood vitamin levels in early pregnancy (Table 9) showed that except for erythrocyte folate, the blood levels we examined were as closely correlated with the dietary intake recorded one year later as with the intake around the time of the blood examination; but all these correlations were so weak as to suggest that dietary data can tell us little about the blood levels in question.

In seeking to explain the weakness of these correlations it must be acknowledged that the estimates of dietary intake would not be expected to reflect totally the true intake during early pregnancy, partly because of limitations in the tables used to convert food to nutrient intake (especially the tables for folate, which do not allow for forms other than "free folate") and partly because diet varies from week to week and may be inaccurately recorded. However, dietary variations over periods of a few weeks tend to be small, according to repeat studies of diet before conception and during the first trimester (1) and during two separate weeks of late pregnancy (15); and even the correlation coefficients we observed between diet in early pregnancy and a year later were of the order of one third to one half (Table 1). Inaccurate recording seems to be less severe when subjects weigh and record their food intake prospectively (as in the present study) than when they are asked to recall what they have eaten (12, 15); and when we compared the findings for all women with those whose diaries were judged to be of particularly high quality, we found that although variations in accuracy could lead to spurious social class differences in recorded diet (Table 3), the correlations between dietary and blood vitamin levels for the "good recorders" were very similar to those for all women (Table 9).

It is therefore difficult to believe that correlations as low as these would have occurred if diet had been the only important source of variation in blood vitamin levels within our study population. It seems more likely that a substantial proportion of the variance of each of these blood levels was attributable to constitutional factors. However, it may be relevant here that the women studied were probably an unusually well-fed and homogeneous group: when the "good recorders" in this London series are compared with Smithells' series of Leeds women (13) in respect of all the dietary variables we examined (apart from folate, for which Smithells gave no figures), a majority of these variables are found to have higher mean levels and lower standard deviations in the London women than in even the social class I women from Leeds. In a less uniformly well-fed group than the one we studied, one would expect dietary factors to contribute more to the variances of the blood vitamin levels. This could well be the situation in south Wales, which might explain why studies there should yield evidence of much stronger associations between diet and neural tube defects (9) and between diet and blood folate levels (8) than our London data would lead one to expect.

Even if dietary data can tell us little in well-nourished communities about maternal blood levels of nutrients during embryonic development, it seems that data on blood levels a year later may sometimes be more informative: for two of the four blood vitamin levels we examined – erythrocyte folate and serum carotenoids – the coefficients of correlation between early preg-

214 *Ian Leck* et al.

nancy and a year later exceeded a half (Table 6). The tendency for low blood levels of folate and carotenoids to persist·which this finding implies was particularly apparent in the four mothers of malformed children in our series (Table 10).

We conclude that biochemical comparisons of mothers of malformed and normal offspring, carried out 1 or 2 years after these offspring passed through embryonic life, are well worth pursuing as a possible means of identifying associations of aetiological significance between maternal nutritional status and malformations. Any such discoveries might well suggest preventive measures, since even if the nutritional abnormalities they incriminated were largely due to constitutional factors as opposed to diet, it might be possible to correct them by dietary supplementation and so to prevent associated malformations.

Acknowledgements

We are deeply grateful to the British Nutrition Foundation for financial support; to Professor D. V. I. Fairweather and his colleagues of the Professorial Obstetric Unit, University College Hospital, London, for access to their patients; to Dr W. T. C. Berry and to Mrs M. Disselduff of the Department of Health and Social Security, and Dr J. P. Greaves of the Ministry of Agriculture, Fisheries and Food, for advice and access to food codes and conversion tables; to Professor W. W. Holland and his colleagues of the Department of Clinical Epidemiology and Social Medicine, St Thomas's Hospital Medical School, especially Mr D. G. Altman, for advice and for converting the dietary diaries to estimates of daily nutrient and food intake; to Ms Angela Cooper of the Department of Medical Statistics, Christie Hospital and Holt Radium Institute, Manchester, and Ms Jock Hua of the Department of Community Medicine, University of Manchester, for other computational assistance; and to all the mothers in the study population for the ways in which they co-operated with us, often at considerable inconvenience to themselves.

References

1. Beal, V. A. (1971). Nutritional studies during pregnancy: I. Changes in intake of calories, carbohydrates, fat, protein, and calcium. *J. Am. Diet. Assoc.* **58**, 312–326.
2. Dacie, J. V. and Lewis, S. M. (1968). "Practical Haematology" 4th edition. Churchill, London.

3. Gal, I., Sharman, I. M. and Pryse-Davies, J. (1972). Vitamin A in relation to human congenital malformations. *Adv. Teratology* **5**, 143–159.
4. Hoffbrand, A. V., Newcombe, F. A. and Mollin, D. L. (1966). Method of assay of red cell folate activity and the value of the assay as a test for folate deficiency. *J. Clin. Path.* **19**, 17–28.
5. Hurdle, A. D. F. (1967). The folate content of a hospital diet. M.D. thesis, University of London.
6. Hurdle, A. D. F., Barton, D. and Searles, I. H. (1968). A method for measuring folate in food and its application to a hospital diet. *Am. J. Clin. Nutrition* **21**, 1202–1207.
7. Hussain, M. A. and Wadsworth, G. R. (1968). Personal communication.
8. Laurence, K. M., James, N. and Campbell, H. (1982). Quality of diet and blood folate concentrations. *Brit. Med. J.* **285**, 216.
9. Laurence, K. M., James, N., Miller, M. and Campbell, H. (1980). Increased risk of recurrence of pregnancies complicated by fetal neural tube defects in mothers receiving poor diets, and possible benefit of dietary counselling. *Brit. Med. J.* **281**, 1592–1594.
10. Leitner, Z. A., Moore, T. and Sharman, I. M. (1960). Vitamin A and vitamin E in human blood: 1. Levels of vitamin A and carotenoids in British men and women, 1948–57. *Brit. J. Nutrition* **14**, 157–169.
11. Office of Population Censuses and Surveys (1970). "Classifcation of Occupations 1970." Her Majesty's Stationery Office, London.
12. Smithells, R. W. (1982). Prevention of neural tube defects by vitamin supplements. This volume, pp. 53–63.
13. Smithells, R. W., Ankers, C., Carver, M. E., Lennon, D., Schorah, C. J. and Sheppard, S. (1977): Maternal nutrition in early pregnancy. *Brit. J. Nutrition* **38**, 497–506.
14. Smithells, R. W., Sheppard, S. and Schorah, C. J. (1976). Vitamin deficiencies and neural tube defects. *Arch. Dis. Child.* **51**, 944–950.
15. Thomson, A. M. (1958). Diet in pregnancy: 1. Dietary survey technique and the nutritive value of diets taken by primigravidae. *Brit. J. Nutrition* **12**, 446–461.
16. Topp, S. G., Cook, J. and Elliott, A. (1972). Measurement of nutritional intake among schoolchildren: aspects of methodology. *Brit. J. Prev. Soc. Med.* **26**, 106–111.
17. Wadsworth, G. R. (1957). Species difference in trapped plasma of the packed red cell column. *Experientia* **13**, 149–150.
18. Waters, A. H. and Mollin, D. L. (1961). Studies on the folic acid activity of human serum. *J. Clin. Path.* **14**, 335–344.
19. Wootton, I. D. P. (1964). "Micro-analysis in Medical Biochemistry", 4th edition. Churchill, London.

Commentary

Chris Schorah: Leck observes only low correlation coefficients between blood levels in early pregnancy and diet at the same time. We have found similar poor correlation between dietary intake and erythrocyte and serum folate, leucocyte vitamin C and erythrocyte riboflavin; $r = 0.21, 0.25, 0.18$ and -0.22; all correlations significant at $P<0.05$ (erythrocyte riboflavin was assessed as a saturation ratio: the correlation has a negative value because increasing values represent decreasing riboflavin status) (5, 1). We can also confirm that folic acid intakes at Leeds, for which we now have figures (1), were poorer than the values found by Leck, as he has already indicated was the case for other vitamins and blood levels of folic acid were lower than in the south. Our means for erythrocyte and serum folate were 228 and 6.3 ng/ml respectively (4) (compare with Leck, Table 10). However, poor correlations between diet and blood concentrations in Leeds, where intakes and body reserves were lower than in the south, questions the suggestion made by Leck that correlation between levels of vitamins in the diet and blood ought to increase as dietary intake becomes less adequate.

Our folate measurements taken during early pregnancy show no seasonal change in erythrocyte folate but a tendency for serum folate to be lowest in April and May (Table 11). In this study the largest seasonal change was found in vitamin C with the lowest concentrations found in late spring, possibly because of consumption of old potatoes low in vitamin C at this time of the year (2). If the seasonal variation in NTD is consistent and does

Table 11. Plasma folic acid concentrations in the first trimester of pregnancy grouped by month when blood sample taken.

| | Plasma folic acid | |
	Mean $\mu g/l$	(number of observations)
January	6.05	50
February	6.59	83
March	5.76	78
April	5.63	79
May	5.82	75
June	6.77	90
July	6.47	69
August	6.46	31
September	6.20	74
October	6.62	61
November	6.58	57
December	7.11	53

Samples were collected April 1970–July 1972; each value therefore represents the average for that month over a 2–3 year period.

coincide with closure of the neural tube during spring, then slight deficiencies of both these vitamins occurring at the same time could lead to greater problems in maintaining the rate of cell division than more marked deficiencies of either vitamin alone. I have considered possible interrelationships of vitamins in my comments on the paper by Laurence.

Leck concludes his appendix by hoping that biochemical measurements in the mothers of malformed and normal children carried out after the fetuses have passed through embryonic life may well give clues to the aetiology of the disease. This may indeed be the case, but our initial findings from Leeds show similar non-pregnant concentrations of blood folic acid and vitamin C in mothers of both malformed and normal offspring (3). Table 12 shows the mean values for serum and erythrocyte folic acid and leucocyte vitamin C in these two groups. Whilst there are no significant differences in the mean values, there are significantly larger proportions of mothers who have had

Table 12. Blood vitamin concentrations in unsupplemented non-pregnant high-risk[a] and low-risk women (mean values and standard deviations).

	High-risk			Low-risk			
	Mean	s.d.	n	Mean	s.d.	n	
Erythrocyte folic acid (ng/ml)	200	125	68	222	100	100	NS[b]
Serum folic acid (ng/ml)	5·9	3·5	64	5·7	2·5	91	NS
Leucocyte vitamin C (μg/ml blood)	2·08	0·85	67	2·19	0·75	70	NS

[a] High-risk; at least one previous NTD affected pregnancy. Low-risk; no previous NTD affected pregnancy. [b] NS not significantly different.

NTD infants compared with those who have not, with erythrocyte folate and leucocyte vitamin C concentrations below the normal range found in healthy adults (Table 13).

However, the differences are small and recent unpublished work from Smithells' laboratory on two women who have had more than one NTD infant has found perfectly normal non-pregnant blood folate levels and a normal serum folic acid rise following an oral folic acid load. Clearly further investigations are required, but initial findings would suggest that if poor folate status is implicated in the aetiology of NTD, then either there are dramatic changes in folate metabolism during pregnancy in women at risk for NTD, or in these conditions the lesion occurs either during placental–fetal transfer of folate or within the fetus.

Ian Leck et al.

Table 13. Number and percentage of unsupplemented non-pregnant high-risk[a] and low-risk women with blood vitamin concentrations on or below the fifth percentile of the normal range for healthy adults.

	5th percentile	High-risk			Low-risk		
Erythrocyte folic acid (ng/ml)	100	16[b]	24	68	7[b]	7	100
Serum folic acid (ng/ml)	2·2	2	3	64	2	2	91
Leucocyte vitamin C (µg/ml blood)	1·35	14[b]	20	67	3[b]	4	70

[a] High-risk; at least one previous NTD affected pregnancy. Low-risk; no previous NTD affected pregnancy. $2 \times 2x^2$ analysis shows significant difference between high- and low-risk values: [b] $P<0·01$.

1. Rogozinski, H., Ankers, C., Lennon, D., Wild, J., Schorah, C. J., Sheppard, S. and Smithells, R. W. (1982). Folate nutrition in early pregnancy. (in preparation).
2. Schorah, C. J., Zemroch, P. J., Sheppard, S. and Smithells, R. W. (1978). Leucocyte ascorbic acid and pregnancy. *Brit. J. Nutr.* **39**, 139.
3. Schorah, C. J., Wild, J., Hartley, R., Sheppard, S. and Smithells, R. W. (1982). The effect of periconceptional supplementation on blood vitamin concentrations in women at recurrence risk for neural tube defect. *Brit. J. Nutr.* (in press).
4. Smithells, R. W., Sheppard, S. and Schorah, C. J. (1976). Vitamin deficiencies and neural tube defects. *Arch. Dis. Child.* **51**, 944.
5. Smithells, R. W., Ankers, C., Carver, M. E., Lennon, D., Schorah, C. J. and Sheppard, S. (1977). Maternal nutrition in early pregnancy. *Brit. J. Nutr.* **38**, 497.

Economic Aspects of the Prevention of Neural Tube Defects

RON AKEHURST

Institute of Social and Economic Research,
University of York, York

Introduction

The main concern of this conference is whether maternal nutrition plays a role in the causation of neural tube defects (NTD) and if so what that role is. Related questions concern what effects intervention, in the form of supplementation of diet or diet counselling, would have on the incidence and birth prevalence of NTD. Resolution of these questions is necessarily prior to tackling the questions of how any service developments aimed at lowering NTD should be designed. However, if conclusive evidence of an ability to affect the incidence of NTD emerges over time, the questions of whether prophylactic programmes should be mounted, how they should be designed and how much they would cost will come to the fore. It is appropriate, therefore, that some consideration of these questions should be undertaken at an early stage.

The role of economics in this issue is not to say how much money should be spent on prophylaxis or what can be afforded. Rather, it is to set out the costs and benefits of alternative programmes of prevention, with the costs and benefits being specified both in financial and non-financial terms. The aim is to clarify the gains, in terms of healthy babies who would otherwise be handicapped, avoidance of abortions etc. (and possible losses too, if diet supplementation has its risks) which can be purchased by various levels of money expenditure and use of real resources under alternative modes of organization.

As far as this author is aware no social science research has been undertaken into the likely costs and benefits of true preventive policies for NTD. Unlike other papers presented here which have reported existing research this paper can do little more than attempt to set out some of the major issues that would have to be resolved if a preventive policy were to be implemented. In effect it sets out an agenda for social science research together with a few sparse results drawn from related work which is relevant.

Alternatives

A number of alternative strategies for improving the periconceptional diet of women have been suggested both by conference participants and elsewhere. These include:

(1) Identifying, contacting and counselling/supplementing women in particularly high risk groups. Those who have already had an NTD child are an obvious target and their sibs may be another.

(2) Increased health education in schools and post school, possibly using women's magazines, radio etc. as an aid to more formal instruction.

(3) Prepregnancy clinics for those planning pregnancies. These would allow diet counselling and supplementation and might incidentally allow a number of other benefits to be reaped, e.g. counselling against smoking and drinking.

(4) Contraceptive pill supplementation to protect unplanned pregnancies due to pill failures. This would involve persuading women to take vitamin pills when oral contraceptives were omitted in each cycle.

(5) Fortification of basic foodstuffs, such as bread. This suggestion is likely to attract opposition in principle as in the case of fluoridation of water supplies. However, the greater the extent to which the alternative proposals are costly and/or ineffective and the more effective is the strategy of fortifying basic foodstuffs, the more likely it is that such opposition would be overcome.

With the exception of the final alternative the main costs of the programmes are unlikely to lie in the price of the vitamin supplements. The vitamin preparations are cheap and if produced on a very large scale would be cheaper still. The major part of the cost is almost certain to be taken up by the infrastructure needed to ensure that women actually get the counselling or diet supplementing tablets, and that once they have received them they do actually change their diet or take the tablets.

How easy it would be to persuade women to participate in, and comply with any dietary supplementation scheme is not clear. Over 50% of women approached declined to participate in Laurence's study (Chapter 4), with a significant level of non-compliance among those who initially agreed to do so. Much better compliance was believed to have been achieved by Smithells (8) using a different approach, but precise levels were unknown. In a review of Canadian experience of nutrition counselling of pregnant women to prevent low-birth-weight babies, Wynn and Wynn (12) noted that 19% of mothers included in a dietary counselling project were "uncooperative". A further 3% were suspected of not giving accurate reports about their changes in dietary habits.

It is not known whether women at low risk of bearing an NTD child would be more or less likely to be compliant than those at high risk. On the one hand low-risk women presumably have less incentive as a consequence of their lower risk status. On the other hand high risk women may contain among their number a greater than average proportion of those who are relatively careless of their own health and that of the unborn child, either because of personality or ignorance.

It is probable for each of the alternative strategies that extra success in modifying the dietary habits of women will only be bought by spending extra money. It is also probable that ever increasing marginal amounts will have to be spent to bring in each extra woman. In economist's terms the marginal costs of achieving compliance are likely to rise with the level of compliance achieved.

Also important would be the risk characteristics of the women "captured" by a scheme. Would particularly risky women be picked up first or last? If the latter is the case then the marginal benefits in terms of reduced incidence of NTD achieved by increasing compliance would also increase in the way in which marginal costs might be expected to increase. Each extra woman brought in would yield a progressively greater expected benefit. How far a programme were taken would thus partly depend on the balance between these marginal costs and benefits.

It is clear that at the moment we have very little idea of the magnitudes of the relevant relationships on either the cost or benefit sides. These relationships would become urgent research topics in the event of the role of maternal diet becoming clear enough to influence health service policy.

Benefits from a Programme of Prevention

The term "benefit" is widely used in this type of context to cover two rather different types of outcome. The first is what may be regarded as the true benefit of a programme of prevention, that is the reduction in distress etc. to those directly involved in the existence of a fetus with NTD. There are the parents and other members of the family who have to cope with abortion, either spontaneous or induced, or the birth of a child with NTD; and the child itself if it survives. The second kind of benefit arises from the fact that avoidance of NTD affected fetuses has resource consequences, i.e. various people have more resources available to them as a consequence. To focus attention on what is really at issue, the prevention of the development of damaged fetuses, and particularly the birth of babies with NTD, it is probably better to treat such resource savings as "negative costs". That is, such benefits should be set off against the direct costs of any programme to provide an estimate of its nett cost.

Estimating the benefits from any preventive programme is complicated by the fact that there are already screening programmes in existence designed to detect NTD fetuses in the womb by use of maternal serum alfafetoprotein (MSAFP) levels, amniotic fluid AFP levels and ultrasonography either singly or in some combination. Thus the estimates made of the benefit from a preventive programme will depend on whether or not the screening programme is continued. In turn, the latter is likely to depend on the expected success of the preventive programme.

The benefits from a preventive programme can be classified as follows:

(1) *Reduction in the distress associated with the births of NTD Children.* The size of this reduction would depend on the existing extent of any screening programmes and their degree of success. Some reduction in NTD births would occur even if all pregnant women were screened, because screening does not detect closed lesions, which have been estimated (7) to account for about 15% of all cases. In addition not all open lesions are detected. There has been some debate recently about how successful MSAFP screening programmes are (1, 9), and there is also the possibility that more effective screening methods based on ultrasonography will supersede serum and amniotic fluid screening (2).

(2) *Reduction in distress due to spontaneous abortions of NTD fetuses.*

(3) *Reduction in distress associated with MSAFP screening, amniocentesis and abortion to the extent that screening becomes unnecessary or no longer detects raised serum AFP.* The major gains here would be

reduction in damage by amniocentesis to otherwise healthy fetuses, estimated (7) at about 25 per 100 000 pregnancies screened, removal of worries caused by false positive screening results, and reduced therapeutic abortions.

(4) *To the extent that screening programmes were dismantled, the saving in the cost of running them.*

(5) *The resources saved as a consequence of healthy rather than NTD children being born.*

The size of gains under headings 1, 2, 3 and 5 above would almost certainly depend on the mode of provision of the preventive service and its scale (and therefore cost), as has already been suggested. The classification and estimation of gains under heading 5 is difficult and contentious and requires a little further discussion.

Resources Saved

Presenting the saving of resources in blanket figures is inevitably somewhat misleading because resources are always gained or lost by somebody and we may as a society be as much interested in *who* gains and loses as in how much. Three groups potentially affected by the introduction of a preventive programme are of particular policy relevance in this instance. The first of these comprises the families directly affected, they are after all the prime object of the policy. The second is the government, which is concerned at the effect a prevention programme would have on its expenditures and revenues. The present government is particularly concerned at effects on its budget for what it sees as overriding macroeconomic reasons. Thus it is conceivable that a policy which implied a sizeable financial gain to society as a whole, but a loss to the Exchequer (particularly in the short term) would be regarded unfavourably by the government. The third group whose gains are of interest we can call "the rest of society", i.e. society less the families directly affected. It is this group which subsidises, by its own reduction in consumption, care for persons handicapped by NTD.

Time and the Estimation of Financial Benefits

A commonly expressed view when preventive programmes are mooted is that they must be "worth it" if only because of all the money that would be saved currently used in caring for sufferers. Governments and other decision-making authorities tend to be less impressed with this argument than the protagonists of prevention. One reason might be scepticism about the effectiveness of a preventive programme and the ability to truly save the "caring" resources. This is a question of specifying intervention – outcome relationships carefully and convincingly, taking into account the difficulties of running a prevention programme in practice. A more fundamental reason relates to the fact that the costs of preventive programmes are incurred immediately while the resource savings only accrue slowly after the passage of years.

Both individuals and governments possess the characteristic known as "time preference". That is they prefer costs in the future to costs now, and benefits now to benefits in the future. This characteristic is quite independent of the presence or absence of inflation. Although the latter may be of importance in some individual instances, it is proper to ignore inflation (to the extent that it affects all prices equally) and to carry out all calculations on a fixed price base. For an explanation and discussion of these issues see Sugden and Williams (10) and Pearce and Nash (6). Time preference is given concrete expression in the form of the "discount rate" which enables future costs and benefits to be scaled down for appropriate comparison with present day costs and benefits. The use of the discount rate renders the present value of future financial benefits progressively smaller the higher the discount rate. Thus very large financial gains twenty years hence become rather small in present value terms when discounted at a discount rate of 5% or more. One hundred pounds in twenty years has a present value of £37·69 when discounted at 5%.

The choice of discount rate is thus very important and what rates shall be used in social decision is in fact a highly contentious issue in economics and government. There is official guidance (4) for decisions that involve public money and this recommends employing a discount rate of 5% in health contexts. There are some good reasons for doubting whether this is the appropriate rate to choose in the case of prevention of NTD births and future research should explore the effects of choosing different rates. However, for the purposes of this paper the 5% rate has been accepted and the figures below are calculated on that basis.

Magnitudes of Potential Financial Savings from a Programme of Prevention of NTD

Two sets of calculations useful for our purposes have been produced relating to financial effects of *screening* for NTD. The first of these, by a DHSS working group (7), looked at the costs *to the health service* of a national screening programme, while the second, by Henderson (3), was concerned with the resource savings *to the community in general* of such a programme. A proper cost benefit study of a programme of prevention of NTD would have to put all costs and cost savings on the same footing, as indicated earlier. However, it may be of value to this conference to have some idea, albeit a rather rough one, of the potential financial impact of a preventive programme.

Resources Released by the Discontinuance of the Current Screening Programme

The resources released here will obviously depend on the size of the present screening programme. The working group reported (ref. 7, table 1A) that 32% of areas undertook screening routinely in 1977 and that 72 909 women were screened. Assuming that the number of pregnancies screened increased in proportion to the number of areas undertaking screening, as reported in Wald *et al.* (11) to 1979 and then remained constant we obtain an estimated annual number of women screened of 105 336. Multiplying this figure by the working group's estimate of the cost per woman screened (ref. 7, table 8C), correcting for the discount rate and updating to November 1981 prices (using the DHSS Hospital and Community Health Expenditure Index) yields an estimate of expenditure on screening of about one million pounds per year. Of course, if more women are being screened the potential savings would be correspondingly larger.

The fact that this level of resources was committed to the screening programme would not necessarily mean that this level would be released by the introduction of a preventive programme. First, the screening programme might not be discontinued. Secondly, even if it were it would, at the very least, take some time to move elsewhere resources that were locked up in manpower and equipment. It is conceivable that no financial saving would in fact be made and simply a higher level of service provided in other areas of ante-natal care.

Resources Released by the Substitution of Healthy for NTD Babies

Henderson (3) has estimated the "excess cost" (ref. 3, Table A7) of a cohort of 100 individuals handicapped by spina bifida over their lifetime making due allowance for survival prospects and discounting the costs. This estimate indicates how much "the rest of society" has to pay to care for and maintain an affected individual, relative to their healthy counterparts. Recalculating

Henderson's figure at the current DHSS recommended discount rate of 5%, and updating the figures to a November 1981 price base yields an estimate of savings of £78 600* per year, per hundred live births of spina bifida infants prevented. Note that achieving these gains depends on lowering birth prevalence rather than incidence of NTD, and that successful screening programmes would lower the potential size of the financial gains.

Conclusions

The research question which comes before any economic analysis is whether, by supplementing or amending the diet of women about the time of pregnancy, we have the ability to reduce the incidence of NTD. If that ability is established, then questions about how best to affect maternal diet, and the level of resources to be committed to doing it, come to the fore. At present we have no knowledge of what the quantitative relationships would be between the mounting of a prevention programme (by whatever means) and its outcome in terms of NTD, abortions etc. Correcting that ignorance is essential for the guidance of policy and depends not only on the resolution of medico-scientific questions but also on the resolution of administrative and economic questions. Social science research has its place in answering the latter.

References

1. Brock, D. J. H. (1982). Impact of maternal serum alpha-fetoprotein screening on antenatal diagnosis. *Brit. med. J.* **285**, 365–367.
2. Harris, R. and Read, A. P. (1981). New uncertainties in prenatal screening for neural tube defect. *Brit. med. J.* **282**, 1416–1418.
3. Henderson, J. B. (1982) An economic appraisal of the benefits of screening for open spina bifida. *Social Science and Medicine* **16**, 545–560.
4. H.M. Treasury (1982). "Investment Appraisal in the Public Sector." HMSO.
5. Laurence, K. M., Campbell, H. and James, N. E. The role of improvement in the maternal diet and preconceptional folic acid supplementation in the prevention of neural tube defects. This volume, pp. 85–107.
6. Pearce, D. W. and Nash, C. A. (1981). "The Social Appraisal of Projects." Macmillan, London.
7. Department of Health and Social Security (1979). Report by the Working Group on Screening for Neural Tube Defects.
8. Smithells, R. W., Sheppard, S., Schorah, C. J., Seller, M. J., Nevin, N. C., Harris, R., Read, A. P. and Fielding, D. W. (1981). Apparent prevention of

* Annual equivalent amortized at 5% over 50 years.

neural tube defects by periconceptional vitamin supplementation. *Arch. Dis. Child.* **56**, 911–918.
9. Standing, S. J., Brindle, M. J., MacDonald, A. P. and Lacey, R. W. (1981). Maternal alpha-fetoprotein screening: two years experience in a low risk district. *Brit. med. J.* **283**, 705–707.
10. Sugden, R. and Williams, A. (1978). "The Principles of Practical Cost-benefit Analysis." Oxford University Press, Oxford.
11. Wald, N. J., Cuckle, H. S. and Harwood, C. A. (1979). Screening for open neural tube defects in England and Wales. *Brit. med. J.* **ii**, 331.
12. Wynn, M. and Wynn, A. (1975). "Nutrition Counselling in the Prevention of Low Birth-Weight." Foundation for Education and Research in Child Bearing, London.

Commentary

John Edwards:

(1) "Savings" in practice mean the diversion of equipment and staff and the consequent "upgrading" of obstetrics and hospital biochemistry. Fortunately all the equipment used (ultrasound, centrifuge, radio-immunoassay devices and computers) are in short supply. The advance in obstetric standards secondary to the greater availability of ultrasound, and the consequent reduction in birth casualties, would be a real saving in terms of looking after handicapped children.

(2) The author does not mention the time scale. The DHSS requested advice from the MRC in 1980. If the trial starts in 1983, and becomes the basis for advice, then a decision on whether second affected children are preventable could be made by 1986 on MRC data. This in no way means that the majority of affected children could have been protected in the same way. At the same rate no decision on this would be likely before 1990. As this matter has not been considered perhaps I could attempt to clarify this unfortunate possibility. Suppose that serum folate, or some similar substance was responsible; we could then envisage the type of distribution and response shown in Fig. 1.

The third distribution is obtained by multiplying the heights of the first two curves for each level of nutrient. We do not know the slopes of these distributions, or the risk of NTD at "saturation" levels of "nutrient". Clearly the incidence cannot be reduced to below this by adding nutrients to the population. There is no way this question can be solved by studying the sub-population selected for high risk so, even if the MRC trial ends up in 1986 with 70:10 for the non-folic and folic groups, it would still be impossible

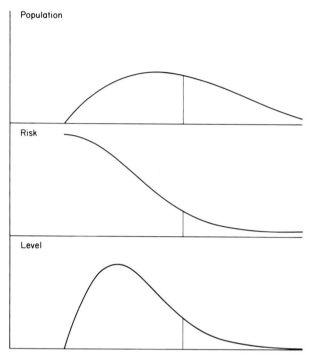

Fig. 1. The upper curve is the distribution of a population of women exposed to a risk of spina bifida which is high at low levels of this hypothetical nutrient. The middle curve shows the risk. The bottom curve, which is the product of the upper two, shows the distribution of mothers with affected children. Supplementation which increased the levels to at least the critical time shown would reduce the incidence of second cases far more than it could reduce the incidence of first cases if applied to the population.

It is known that the risk for populations with 0, 1 and 2 affected children varies by a factor of over 100 to 1. That is no reason to postulate any fetus is at zero risk.

to justify supplementing populations, women, married women, or any other subgroup except those defined by having had an affected child.

The question asked by the DHSS of the MRC, whose economic consequences are explored in this paper, presumably related to supplementing the majority of pregnancies. The question the MRC trial is designed to answer is the quite different one relating to a subgroup of less than 1% of women selected by manifestation of fetal disease.

It might be considered wise to answer the supplementary question first, and, in 1980, this was an open question, in the sense of a substantial degree of expert doubt.

Chris Schorer: I think, interesting though Akehurst's projections are, that this paper merely illustrates the thinking of an economist in a socio-medical context. The absence of hard fact concerning the efficacy of nutritional prevention of NTD makes it impossible for Akehurst to be specific and the paper – through no fault of the authors – is thus of limited value.

I am sorry that Akehurst has not mentioned the importance of press and public opinion in his economic equation (compare the action being contemplated concerning the removal of lead from petrol).

Possible Prevention of Neural Tube Defects by Vitamin Supplementation

NICHOLAS WALD

The Radcliffe Infirmary,
Oxford

The Central Issue

The central issue is whether vitamin supplementation can prevent fetal neural tube defects. In assessing the relevant evidence it is more important to see whether the available data can withstand specific attempts at refutation than it is to see whether they are *consistent* with the hypothesis. There is probably no disagreement that there are data consistent with the hypothesis, namely those from *in vitro* experiments using whole embryo cultures (see Beck's paper), from *in vivo* experiments performed on rats and mice (see Seller's paper), and from observational studies in humans both with respect to the identification of nutritional deficiencies by dietary assessment and blood measurements (see Laurence's and Smithells' papers).

These data do not, however, provide good evidence that vitamin supplementation can prevent neural tube defects. The *in vitro* experiments using whole embryo cultures are still only at an early stage, and in the one experiment described in which folate deficiency was investigated (paper by

Cockroft (1) cited in Beck's paper) no failure of neural tube defect closure was apparent. In the animal experiments, folate deficiency has not been shown to produce neural tube defect formation unless also accompanied by the use of folate antagonists and the lesions produced are relatively non-specific including several different types of malformation. The human evidence is also non-specific since nutritional deficiency in one substance is highly correlated with deficiencies in other substances, as well as with other non-nutritional factors, such as level of disposable income and quality of housing.

The most promising results concerning vitamin supplementation in the prevention of neural tube defects arise from the two recent human intervention studies.

The Intervention Study Performed by Smithells and his Colleagues

While it is most unlikely that the results of the study by Smithells and his colleagues (7, 8) arose by chance (see Table 1), the conclusion that it was the multivitamin administration that led to the reduction in the incidence of neural tube defects rests on the assumption that, in the absence of vitamin supplementation, the vitamin supplemented group and the control group were equally at risk of having an affected fetus (or if they were not, the difference was significantly smaller than the difference observed). There is, however, evidence to show that this assumption cannot be made. For example, the group of women who selected themselves for supplementation included a relatively low proportion of (a) women of low social class (56% compared with 69% in the unsupplemented group (Table 2)), and (b) women who had a miscarriage in the immediately previous pregnancy (8% compared with 17% in the unsupplemented group (Table 3)). Since low

Table 1. Outcome According to Treatment Received.

Outcome	Treatment received Fully supplemented	Unsupplemented	Total
NTD	3	23	26
Not NTD	394	470	864
Total	397	493	890

Relative risk of NTD if unsupplemented = 6·48. (Taken from refs 7 and 8).

Table 2. Treatment Group According to Social Class.

| Social class | Treatment group | | |
	Fully supplemented	Unsupplemented	Total
High[a]	86	87	173
Low[b]	110	191	301
Total	196	278	474

[a] High = I, II, III non-manual. [b] Low = III manual, IV, V. Relative risk of being supplemented if high social class = 1·72 (taken from Table 4 in ref. 7).

social class and previous miscarriage are risk factors for neural tube defects (with relative risks of 3·7 and 1·6 respectively, see Tables 4 and 5), the women who had selected themselves for treatment were at relatively low risk of having a fetal neural tube defect.

Allowing for the confounding effects of social class and immediately previous miscarriage would have reduced the strength of the association between supplementation and low risk of neural tube defect. Such a reduction due to confounding from just two factors which happened to have been estimated in the study, illustrates the possibility that had other relevant factors been estimated, allowance for them might have actually abolished the association, and hence any claim that vitamin supplementation prevents neural tube defects. It is also likely that, had those social class factors which were relevant to the risk of having neural tube defects been measured more precisely than by simply categorizing women according to their husband's occupation (which is the basis of social class coding), adjusting for these factors would reduce still further the strength of the association between supplementation and risk of neural tube defects.

Table 3. Treatment Group According to Outcome of Previous Pregnancy.

| Outcome of previous pregnancy | Treatment group | | |
	Fully supplemented	Unsupplemented	Total
Miscarriage	17	51	68
Not a Miscarriage	183	249	432
Total	200	300	500

Relative risk of being unsupplemented if previous pregnancy was a miscarriage = 2·20. (taken from Table 5 in ref. 7).

Table 4. Outcome According to Social Class.

Social class	Outcome NTD	Not NTD	Total
High[a]	2	194	196
Low[b]	12	312	324
Total	14	506	520

[a] High = I, II, III non-manual. [b] Low = III manual, IV, V and un-employed. Relative risk of NTD outcome if low social class = 3·73 (taken from Table 4 in ref. 7).

A particularly relevant study showing how self selection to a pill-taking therapeutic regime can produce strikingly spurious results is provided by the Report of the Coronary Drug Project group published in 1980 (2). The key results are shown in Table 6. Subjects who were regarded as being compliant (taking at least 80% of their pills) had a 15% five year mortality compared with a 25% mortality among those who were not compliant – the treatment under study being clofibrate, a cholesterol-lowering drug. The results would have suggested that clofibrate could reduce mortality from coronary heart disease by 40% were it not for the fact that the study was a randomized placebo controlled investigation and the corresponding mortality among subjects who did and did not comply in the *placebo* group was 15% and 28% – an apparent reduction of 46%! The correct analysis of the study showed that the group allocated to clofibrate had an 18% mortality – virtually the same as that observed in the group allocated to the placebo (19% mortality). An additional point of importance in this study is that, in spite of estimating a large number of possible confounding factors, it would not have been possible to have made any allowance for the self-selection bias since, among

Table 5. Outcome of Current Pregnancy (NTD or Non-NTD) According to Outcome of Previous Pregnancy.

Outcome	Outcome of previous pregnancy Miscarriage	Not a miscarriage	Total
NTD	74	211	285
Not NTD	24	109	133
Total	98	320	418

Relative risk of NTD outcome if previous pregnancy was a miscarriage = 1·59. (Taken from ref. 3).

Table 6. The Coronary Drug Project: Five year mortality in patients given clofibrate or placebo according to compliance with the treatment.

Compliance	Clofibrate		Placebo	
	No. of patients	Five year mortality	No. of patients	Five year mortality
<80%	357	25% ⎫	882	28% ⎫
		⎬ *		⎬ *
≥80%	708	15% ⎭	1813	15% ⎭
Total	1065	18%	2695	19%

(Taken from ref. 2). (*$P<0.001$.)

subjects allocated to clofibrate, those who took it did not differ significantly from those who did not in respect of a wide variety of factors. The fact that specific confounding factors could be identified in the study performed by Smithells and his colleagues suggests that the overall effect of self-selection in that study may have been greater than was found to be the case in the coronary heart disease study.

It is worth noting that there are documented examples of uncontrolled or poorly controlled intervention studies that initially suggested quite striking therapeutic benefits, but which, later, after the conduct of properly controlled investigations, yielded results that showed that the benefit was less than was first expected, or even non-existent. The paper by Sacks and Chalmers (6) gives several examples.

There is, to my knowledge, only one piece of evidence to suggest that the effects of self-selection in the study of Smithells and his colleagues may not have been strong. This comes from the study of neural tube defect prevention by potato avoidance (see paper by Nevin) where women who complied with the advice to avoid potatoes did not have a low risk recurrence, suggesting that women who comply with this advice are not self-selected from a low risk group. If the factors which influence compliance are similar for a vitamin pill regime and a potato avoidance regime then this would lend weight to the view that the self-selection explanation for the results of the vitamin supplementation study could be rejected, leaving one with the alternative explanation, namely that the vitamins were therapeutically active. However, it is not clear whether the self-selection factors which influence taking pills regularly in the absence of symptoms are the same (in nature and extent) as those affecting the avoidance of potatoes. Also the results were based on small numbers; there were only two neural tube defect pregnancies (out of 23) among the women on the potato-free diet.

In summary, I believe we must conclude that self-selection did introduce at least *some* bias into the study performed by Smithells and his colleagues. We cannot say, however, that bias explains all the results; there may have also been a direct therapeutic effect of the vitamins. The problem is that it is not possible to disentangle the extent to which self-selection or therapeutic effect, if any, accounted for the observed results.

The Intervention Study Performed by Laurence and his Colleagues (4)

The study of folic acid supplementation is subject to the same possible self-selection bias described above when the data are analysed according to whether the women took the pills they were given. However, the study was a double-blind randomized trial and when the results were analysed according to the group to which the women were allocated, the criticism of the study is not one of design but simply that the study was too small. Two out of 60 women allocated to the folic acid group had fetal neural-tube defects compared with 4 out of 63 allocated to the placebo group. The results are obviously consistent with a 50% reduction in risk of fetal neural-tube defects attributable to folic acid supplementation, although they could easily have been due to chance. If a larger number of women had been recruited to the study, the matter could have been resolved.

Summary of the Two Intervention Studies

The study by Smithells and his colleagues (7, 8) was large enough but inadequately controlled and, to some extent, biased. The study by Laurence and his colleagues (4) was unbiased but too small. The case for vitamin supplementation being an effective method of preventing neural tube defects is therefore weak and we are left in considerable scientific doubt as to whether there is a specific and direct effect of either folic acid or other vitamin supplementation in preventing neural tube defects.

Possible Adverse Effects Associated with Vitamin Supplementation

It has been argued that it is unimportant whether the vitamin supplementation is proven to be effective, since the pills are bound to be safe; there is therefore no reason not automatically to offer supplementation and give women the "benefit" of the doubt. Regrettably, however, there are many examples of medical treatments that were at one time thought to be completely safe but later were shown to produce harmful effects, some of them serious. For example, the use of vitamin D to prevent rickets led to the production of hypercalcaemia and its serious consequences. Even in modest doses, a small group of children with vitamin D sensitivity can suffer adverse effects. Another example is the use of oxygen in the treatment of premature babies. This is a particularly relevant example, since at one time oxygen was regarded as being so safe that it was impossible to give too much – a view which was reversed only after the realization that a number of infants became blind due to retrolental fibroplasia. The third example is the administration of diethylstilboestrol during pregnancy to prevent recurrent miscarriage. Again it was argued that female sex hormones were "normal" and one was simply supplementing a group who may have been deficient. Later it emerged that not only was the treatment ineffective, but it also caused vaginal cancer in the daughters of the treated women. (The last two examples have been cited in this context by Paul Meier (5)).

The fact that all the vitamins in question, except folic acid in unusual doses, can be obtained without prescription in the UK, does not mean that the regular administration of extra vitamins, even in doses approximating to the recommended daily allowances, will not be associated with some adverse effect when administered in well nourished communities. Some mothers or fetuses may show particular sensitivity to certain vitamins, and others who might already be taking large quantities, will consume even more as a result of the supplementation. In addition, one cannot exclude the possibility of therapeutic abuse in which women, or perhaps their children, will consume excessive doses of the vitamins. Of course this is a potential hazard with all medication, but it is none the less a factor which needs to be taken into account when assessing the overall hazards and benefits of the treatment regime.

A problem associated with the evaluation of a new treatment regime is that while the expected benefit is specific and often inferred on the basis of previous uncontrolled experiments, the possibility of harm remains hypothetical until someone suspects a specific abnormality associated with the treatment. This, of course, should not be taken to mean that no hazard in fact exists. In general the evaluation of the efficacy of a treatment regime should also attempt to identify possible hazards. However, in this particular example there is a difficulty because a study capable of detecting a 50% reduction in the risk of neural tube defects associated with vitamin supplementation among women who have already had at least one affected infant, will not be statistically powerful enough to detect adverse effects associated with an absolute increase in risk of, say, a serious malformation of about 2 per 1000 – equivalent to increasing the background risk of many serious malformations two or three-fold. (In assessing the likely benefit in relation to the possible hazard it should be borne in mind that about 90% of neural tube defects can be detected antenatally, but any abnormality caused by the vitamin supplementation may not.) Perhaps the sensible course of action is to design unbiased studies capable of assessing whether vitamin supplementation is effective, and if so, the approximate magnitude of the effect, while at the same time collecting sufficient identifying information of the children born to the treated women so that if the treatment is found to be effective, the children can be followed up for the closer scrutiny of adverse effects – perhaps combining the results of several studies in order to obtain the statistical power necessary for the detection of the sort of risks which might be expected.

The Future

Two types of study can help establish whether vitamin supplementation can reduce the risk of neural tube defects. First, large randomized studies, which would be unbiased and therefore resolve the principal objection to the existing studies. Unfortunately reporting of the subject in the media may have led the public into believing that the vitamins are beneficial, and in spite of the uncertain scientific position this has almost certainly made it more difficult to carry out the necessary randomized studies. This itself raises an issue about the dangers of publicity prior to the launching of a clinical trial which may prevent the trial taking place, and hence leave unresolved an important medical issue. This issue, which affects clinical trials in general, needs further general discussion.

The second method of evaluating the efficacy of vitamin supplementation would be a "total ascertainment" study, in which all eligible patients within a geographical area are defined, the treatment offered to all, and an attempt made to reach 100% compliance. Then the frequency of neural tube defects would be assessed in the total group (supplemented *and* unsupplemented) – the results being compared with those during an earlier period (historical controls) or those from another geographical area (geographical controls). This approach is much less satisfactory than the randomized design, since unless the effect of treatment is dramatic it is possible that any differences observed were due to factors other than the treatment itself, e.g. differences in the risk of neural tube defects over time or between different geographical areas.

It is perhaps being wise after the event to point out that the present problem would not have arisen if the ethical committees which considered the study performed by Smithells and his colleagues (7, 8) had not decided against a randomized study, or if the investigators had challenged the decision and persisted in their view that a randomized design was advisable. None the less there is undoubtedly a lesson to be learned. Ethical committees need to be more accountable (perhaps publishing, in an annual report, their decisions and reasons for refusal) and investigators must be prepared to press their case more strongly if they feel it is a correct one, and have the right of appeal.

References

1. Cockroft, D. L. (1979). Nutrient requirements of rat embryos undergoing organogenesis *in vitro. J. Reproduct. Fertil.* **57**, 505–10.
2. The Coronary Drug Project Research Group. (1980). Influence of adherence to treatment and response of cholesterol on mortality in the Coronary Drug Project. *N. Eng. J. Med.* **303**, 1038–41.
3. Laurence, K. M. and Roberts, C. J. (1977). Spina bifida and anencephaly: are miscarriages a possible cause? *Brit. med. J.* **2**, 361.
4. Laurence, K. M., James, N., Miller, M. H., Tennant, G. B. and Campbell, H. (1981). Double-blind randomised controlled trial of folate treatment before conception to prevent recurrence of neural tube defects. *Brit. Med. J.* **282**, 1509–11.
5. Meier, P. (1982). Vitamins to prevent neural tube defects. *Lancet* i, 859.
6. Sacks, H., Chalmers, T. C. and Smith, H. (1982). Randomised versus historical controls for clinical trials. *Am. J. Med.* **72**, 233–40.
7. Smithells, R. W., Shepherd, S., Schorah, C. J., Seller, M. J., Nevin, N. C., Harris, R., Read, A. P. and Fielding, D. W. (1981). Apparent prevention of neural tube defects by vitamin supplementation. *Arch. Dis. Child.* **56**, 911–18.
8. Smithells, R. W., Shepherd, S., Schorah, C. J., Seller, M. J., Nevin, N. C., Harris, R., Read, A. P., Fielding, D. W. and Walker, S. (1981). Vitamin supplementation and neural tube defects. *Lancet* ii, 1424–5.

Critical Glossary

The following terms were found to require definition during discussion at the Workshop:

Alphafetoprotein. A fetal homologue of albumin, produced in very small amounts after mid-pregnancy. (J.H.E.)

Anencephaly. A failure of the cranium to form, characterized by the absence of skull vault and brain. The eyes are usually proptosed but the remainder of the face is normal. (N.C.N.) See also *Neural Tube Defect* (J.H.E.)

Congenital. Evident at birth. (J.H.E.)

Craniorhhachischis. A failure of the whole neural tube to close and results in anencephaly and a completely open spine. (N.C.N.) See also *Neural Tube Defect* (J.H.E.)

Endephalocoele. A defect in the cranium usually the occipital region through which meninges and brain tissue protrude. Usually covered with skin. (N.C.N.)

Enrichment. See Fortification.

Folic Acid. Generic descriptor for the different forms of the naturally occurring vitamin. These are pteroylmonoglutamate and the pteroylpolyglutamates from two to eight glutamate residues. In addition the vitamin is found in reduced form (either as di- or tetrahydropteroylglutamates) and as methyl and formyl derivatives in both plant and animal foods (IUNS Committee on Nomenclature, Nutr. Abs. Rev. A., 1978, 48, 831). (D.J.N.)

Folic acid (Fig. 1) is a substituted pterin residue linked through a methylene bridge to para-aminobenzoic acid which in turn is joined through a peptide bond to a glutamic acid residue. This is folic acid or pteroylglutamic acid, but there are many different biologically active derivatives of this compound which vary in:

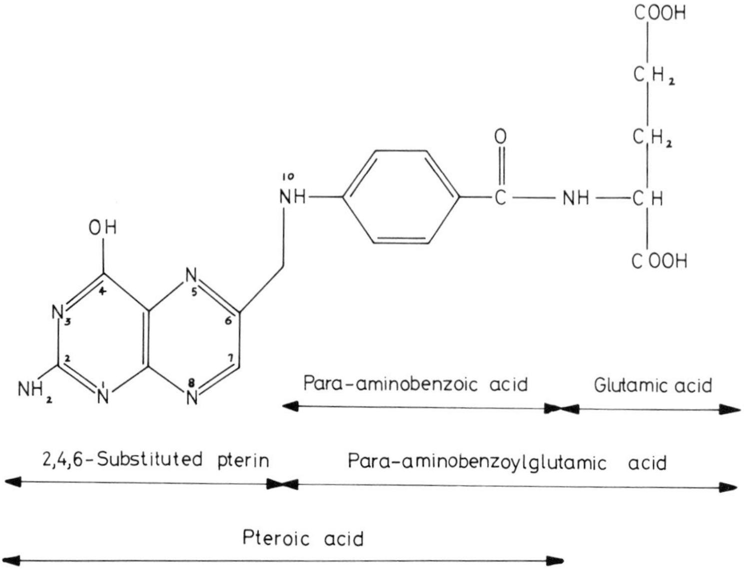

Fig. 1. The structural formula of folic acid (Pteroylglutamic acid).

(1) The degree of reduction of the pterin ring at positions 5, 6, 7 and 8 producing dihydro- and tetrahydrofolic acids (di- and tetrahydro-pteroyl glutamates).

(2) The presence of a variety of one carbon substituents linked between position 5 on the pterin residue and 10 on the *p*-aminobenzoic acid. Such substituents differ in their state of oxidation from the fully reduced methyl through to the oxidized formate.

(3) The number of glutamic acid residues linked through peptide bonds to form polyglutamate chains of different lengths.

Dietary folates are a complex mixture of many of these derivatives of folic acid. Folic acid in supplements however, is in the oxidized, non-substituted monoglutamate form (the structure in Fig. 1), but this only comprises about 1% of the folate in the average diet. For simplicity, we will use folic acid or folate as a general term to cover the many forms of the vitamin in foods, in blood and in metabolism, and reserve the name folate monoglutamate for the vitamin in tablet form, such as Pregnavite forte F®. (C.J.S.)

Fortification. Is used interchangeably with *Enrichment*, to mean the addition of a nutrient that was not present in the food, or present in small amounts only. The proposal that folic acid might be added to white flour for bread making is not a viable one. The compulsory enrichment of white flour with vitamins and minerals is to be discontinued in the near future. (DHSS Report on Health and Social Subjects No. 23. Nutritional Aspects of Bread and Flour, 1981. HMSO, London.) (D.J.N.)

Genetic. Related to the genetic material acquired at conception. (J.H.E.)

Incidence. This should be reserved for the proportion of those at risk of a disorder who develop it, which in the case of neural tube defects means the proportion of embryos alive at the age when these malformations arise who are affected. (See *Prevalence.*) (I.L.)

Malformation. An error in development evident on gross inspection. (J.H.E.)

Neural Tube Defect. A general term to include lesions which result from failure of the neural tube to close. These include anencephalus, craniorrachischisis, spina bifida, meningocoele, meningomyelocoele, myelocoele and encephalocoele. (N.C.N.)

A term used to describe defects arising from defective closing of the neural tube, especially at its ends. Primary hydrocephalus, although often due to defective patency, is usually excluded. Deficits of the lower end lead to spina bifida, myelocoele and meningomyelocoele which are terms referring to the degree of herniation. If the opening, or hernial sac, is covered with skin, the lesion is termed "closed". These lesions, which do not usually lead to severe consequences, cannot be detected by the transudation of AFP (alphafetoprotein *q.v.*). At the front, herniation of the brain is referred to as *exencephaly*; virtual absence of the brain (which may follow exencephaly and necrosis) is *anencephaly*; and absence of the brain accompanied by absence of the spinal cord with an open bony channel is *craniorrhacischisis.* (J.H.E.)

Prevalence. This is used as shorthand for the prevalence of malformations at birth, i.e. the proportion of children born (including stillbirths) who are affected. (See *Incidence.*) (I.L.)

Spina Bifida. This is due to a failure of closure of the vertebral arches. It is characterized by a protrusion of meninges (meningocoele) or of both meninges and nerve tissue (meningomyelocoele). (N.C.N.)

Spina Bifida Occulta. This is the failure of the vertebral arch to close. This may be associated with a sinus, tuft of hair or haemangioma in lumbosacral region (N.C.N.)

Index